Management of Heart Failure

Second Edition

James B. Young, MD
Medical Director,
Kaufman Center for Heart Failure
Chairman and Professor,
Division of Medicine
Cleveland Clinic Foundation
Lerner College of Medicine of
Case Western Reserve University

Roger M. Mills, MD
Professor of Medicine
Cleveland Clinic Foundation
Lerner College of Medicine of
Case Western Reserve University
Cleveland, Ohio

PROFESSIONAL
COMMUNICATIONS, INC.

Professional Communications, Inc.
A Medical Publishing Company

Marketing Office:
400 Center Bay Drive
West Islip, NY 11795
(t) 631/661-2852
(f) 631/661-2167

Editorial Office:
PO Box 10
Caddo, OK 74729-0010
(t) 580/367-9838
(f) 580/367-9989

For orders only, please call
1-800-337-9838

or visit our website at
www.pcibooks.com

ISBN: 1-884735-90-8

Printed in the United States of America

DISCLAIMER

This text is printed on recycled paper.

DEDICATION

To Katherine, Cody, and BeauZeau (RMM) and Claire, Joey, Jamie, Becky, and Chris × 2 (JBY) with love and appreciation.

ACKNOWLEDGMENT

The authors would like to thank Nancy Albert, RN, MSN, for her commitment to bettering the lives of heart failure patients. Ms. Albert is the principal designer of many heart failure management algorithms seen in this text. We also would be lost without the secretarial skills of Ms. Lisa Paciorek, the editorial patience of Malcolm Beasley and Phyllis Freeny, and the graphic expertise of Nikki D. Merrill.

TABLE OF CONTENTS

TABLES

Introduction

Heart failure (HF) has become epidemic. The aging of the post–World War II "Baby Boom" generation will soon further swell the number of HF patients. According to the American Heart Association's Heart and Stroke Facts, almost five million patients have congestive heart failure (CHF) in the United States, with perhaps as many as a half-million individuals developing symptomatic HF each year. Framingham databases estimate that we have a one in five chance of developing HF in our lifetime. These figures are clearly underestimates since they rely on making a diagnosis of significantly symptomatic CHF that is, in reality, only a small portion of the overall ventricular dysfunction and HF problem.

The incidence of HF more than doubles with each decade after the age of 45, and approximately 35% of all new HF diagnoses result in hospitalization in the subsequent 12 months. Patients with HF comprise the most expensive Medicare diagnosis-related group, with an average length of hospital stay ranging from 5 to 10 days and average costs calculated to be between $7,000 and $15,000. Primary care physicians treat the vast majority of these patients, predominantly in outpatient settings.

Three years ago, we completed the first edition of this text as a practical guide to help clinicians understand the most contemporary evidence-based concepts of HF diagnosis and treatment. In the brief interval between editions, HF diagnosis and management have advanced impressively. The introduction and widespread acceptance of the B-type natriuretic peptide (BNP) assay has refined both diagnosis and management. Nesiritide, the first new parenteral agent approved for HF in over a decade, has claimed an important place in the drug armamentarium for acutely decompensated patients. Evidence-based indications for carvedilol have expanded. New and even more impressive data regarding β-blockers in general have been published. Important new clinical trials have documented roles for candesartan, an angiotensin receptor blocker, and eplerenone, an aldosterone antagonist, in chronic management. New interest has emerged with respect to treating diabetes and anemia in patients with HF. A series of arrhythmia management device trials has firmly established the lifesaving role of implantable defibrillators, and data are rapidly accruing to support cardiac resynchronization device therapy for appropriate patients. And, for the first time, a well-conducted clinical trial has shown improved outcomes for end-stage patients receiving left ventricular assist devices.

Clinicians who manage HF patients have a variety of guidelines to suggest evidence-based "best practice," but enormous challenges remain. Even in the best of circumstances, a complete and accurate diagnosis may be difficult to document. Treatment requires complex polypharmacy and often sophisticated device implantation and follow-up. Savvy clinicians still do well, but learning the "tricks of the trade" is difficult.

This revised text provides a quick reference for clarification of important issues and concepts. The text, although expanded, remains lean and heavily supplemented by tables and figures. We have provided extensive flow diagrams to suggest methods of handling common problems. Chapter 5, *Clinical Trials Shaping Heart Failure Therapeutics*, includes a comprehensive survey of virtually all significant clinical trials that have shaped our treatment approach in a reference table organized according to the trial acronyms. Although we have added a number of citations, the references emphasize material critical to understanding data from clinical trials. For all health care providers dealing with HF patients, these guidelines, flowcharts, and care pathways should help to implement evidence-based current standards of care. Finally, in those situations where no clinical trial evidence points the way, we have offered insights gleaned from our HF practice in the hope that they may help.

We appreciate the support and occasional prodding of our editor, Malcolm Beasley, who encouraged us to produce this second edition. With deep gratitude, we acknowledge the help of Nikki Merrill. Without her production talents and patience, this book would never have come to press.

JBY/RMM
Cleveland, Ohio
April 2004

1
Definition and Epidemiology

Definition

The past century has seen great changes in our understanding of heart failure (HF).[15,57,63,318] **Table 1.1** summarizes how this understanding has evolved and impacted therapeutic strategies. HF was first considered a dropsical condition with generalized edema from fluid retention. After the link to myocardial and circulatory failure was clarified, primitive approaches focused primarily on herbal diuretics, lymphatic and thoracic or abdominal cavity drainage, and "foxglove tea." A focus on pump inadequacy as a prime HF mechanism forced attention to the use of more sophisticated cardiac glycoside preparations and alternative inotropic therapies. This approach has culminated in cardiac transplantation and mechanical circulatory assist devices or artificial hearts for end-stage HF.

The knowledge that ventricular hypertrophy is a component of cardiac decompensation linked HF and hypertension. Early treatment may prevent development of left ventricular dysfunction (LVD) and forestall its progression. The new focus on circulatory dysfunction led to use of drugs other than diuretics and inotropes; ultimately, the importance of vasodilating agents in HF emerged. More recently, clarification of the endocrine and inflammatory pathophysiologic responses to HF gave rise to the use of neurohormonal blocking agents to attenuate HF.

The contemporary definition of HF is complicated. HF is best understood as a milieu of cardiac pump dysfunction (systolic and/or diastolic), myocardial remod-

17

TABLE 1.1 — HOW INSIGHT INTO HEART FAILURE HAS IMPACTED TREATMENT

- Heart failure (HF) is a dropsical condition with generalized edema from fluid retention:
  - Primitive diuretic therapies
  - Lymphatic drainage tubes
  - Thoracic/abdominal cavity drainage
  - "Foxglove" tea
- HF is due to central cardiac pump inadequacy:
  - Cardiac glycoside preparations
  - Alternative inotropic therapies
  - Cardiac transplantation
  - Mechanical ventricular assist devices/total artificial hearts
- HF is precipitated by decompensated ventricular hypertrophy:
  - Antihypertensive therapy
  - Surgical repair of valvular defects causing pressure/volume overloads
- HF is due to circulatory dysfunction:
  - Vasodilator therapy to improve peripheral organ flow and perfusion
- HF is an endocrinopathy:
  - Angiotensin-converting enzyme inhibitor (ACEI) therapy
  - Angiotensin II receptor blockade (ARB)
  - β-Blocker prescription
  - Aldosterone antagonists
- HF is a fever:
  - Cytokine modulating agents
- HF is a complicated milieu of pump dysfunction, myocardial remodeling (ventricular hypertrophy and chamber dilation), and hormonal, cytokine, and neuroregulatory perturbation, with subsequent circulatory insufficiency:
  - ACEI
  - ARB
  - β-Blocker therapy
  - Digoxin therapy
  - Diuretic therapy
  - Aldosterone antagonist
  - Surgical therapies (revascularization, ventricular remodeling, valve repair, mechanical circulatory support, transplantation)

eling (ventricular hypertrophy and/or chamber dilation), and hormonal, cytokine, and neuroregulatory disturbances, with subsequent circulatory insufficiency. Structural cardiac remodeling is also a component of the syndrome, as are arrhythmias.

Because many different diseases can cause myocardial injury with subsequent acute or chronic dysfunction, prevention of injury is paramount. Treating illnesses that may precipitate HF should be given high priority. Because myocyte passive tension and workloads increase in the remodeled heart, reducing preload and afterload will diminish myocardial wall stress and allow beneficial deremodeling of the heart. Since the myocardial interstitium contributes to diastolic dysfunction (the matrix stiffens) and this seems tied to myocardial fibrosis resulting from injury and inflammation, newer treatments have focused on modifying inflammation and preventing remodeling. Reduced peripheral organ blood flow (both at rest and during exercise) is detrimental. Some HF therapies, particularly those given during acute decompensation and/or cardiogenic shock, are designed to increase cardiac output and organ perfusion (as well as decrease cardiac filling pressures). Adverse humoral factors (the endocrinopathy of HF) can be blocked utilizing angiotensin-converting enzyme inhibitors, angiotensin II receptor blocking agents, β-adrenergic blockers, and aldosterone antagonists. Representative agents from these drug classes are now used routinely in HF patients. Surgical procedures can partially reverse detrimental remodeling associated with valvular insufficiency or the globular scarred ventricle commonly seen after myocardial infarction.

Patients with HF may present without symptoms or suffer from a variety of fatigue, dyspnea, or edematous states that fluctuate in severity based on treatment, diet, physical conditioning, and diseases precipitating the syndrome in the first place. In addition to making the appropriate diagnosis, clinicians are charged with designing therapies based on the syndrome's severity. This includes starting treatment protocols for asymptomatic ventricular dysfunction in an attempt to prevent deterioration to a frank congestive state. Patients should be made euvolemic and hemodynamics optimized (normalized) while interventions are used to attenuate inflammation and neurohormonal activation.

The clinical availability of B-type natriuretic peptide (BNP) assays has dramatically improved evaluation and management of HF patients. In most patients, but not all, BNP levels mirror the degree of neurohormonal activation and concomitant volume overload. In the diagnostic evaluation of acutely dyspneic patients, BNP levels help focus attention on either cardiac or noncardiac pathology contributing to the complaints. In long-term management of patients with chronic HF, BNP levels offer important prognostic data and may even be useful in titrating drug therapy to individual needs.

The clinical spectrum of HF is wide. **Table 1.2** compares patients presenting with acute HF, decompensated chronic HF, and stable chronic HF. The patient presenting with acute dyspnea syndromes or cardiogenic shock often has pulmonary edema. Peripheral edema is generally rare, and weight gain often has not occurred. Cardiomegaly may not be present, and patients can present with relatively normal LV ejection fraction. Diastolic dysfunction is extremely important in the severely hypertensive patient and may precipitate the sudden onset of pulmonary edema ("flash" pulmonary edema). Acute severe ischemia and acute mitral or aortic regurgitation are also common causes of flash pulmonary edema. In contrast, patients with decompensated chronic HF generally have systolic LVD, with worsening congestive states emerging slowly, with markedly increased total body volume resulting in pulmonary congestion and peripheral edema.

However, acute pulmonary edema is actually rare in these patients despite an increase in total body salt and water load.

Recognizing the different stages of HF is important because treatment strategies differ depending on any given patient's presentation. **Figure 1.1** emphasizes that these presentations can be interchangeable. As shown in this figure, patients with HF appear in a variety of manners and can have many different long-term courses. Some patients remain asymptomatic for long periods after development of LVD; others simply experience sudden cardiac death without preceding congestive states. Some slowly deteriorate with a steady downhill course and progressively worsening organ congestion. Many patients initially become quite ill with congestive heart failure (CHF) but can be treated effectively so that exercise tolerance improves and volume overload dissipates.

Table 1.3 summarizes common hemodynamic patterns noted in patients undergoing right-heart catheterization studies. Frequently, patients with significant HF have depressed cardiac output (at least with exercise), and those presenting with congestion have elevated right atrial, pulmonary capillary wedge, and pulmonary artery pressures. Rarely, high cardiac output patients with severe anemia or arteriovenous fistulae can develop profound CHF. Treatment of these different HF states is often based on correction of abnormal hemodynamics.

Epidemiology

Table 1.4 summarizes the demographics and statistics regarding HF.[312,316] Four to five million Americans are believed to have symptomatic CHF, with fifteen million patients affected worldwide. In the United States in 1990, there were 700,000 hospital discharges with a primary diagnosis of HF, a fourfold in-

Feature	Acute Heart Failure	Decompensated Chronic Heart Failure	Stable Chronic Heart Failure
Symptom severity	Marked	Marked	Mild to moderate
Pulmonary edema	Frequent	Frequent	Rare
Peripheral edema	Rare	Frequent	Mild
Weight gain	None to mild	Marked	Frequent fluctuations
Total body volume	No change or mild increase	Markedly increased	Moderately increased
Cardiomegaly	Uncommon	Usual	Common
LV systolic function	Variably depressed (diastolic dysfunction important)	Reduced	Markedly reduced
Wall stress	Elevated	Markedly elevated	Mild to markedly elevated
Activation of sympathetic nervous system	Marked	Marked	Mild to marked

TABLE 1.2 — COMPARISON OF ACUTE, DECOMPENSATED, AND STABLE CHRONIC HEART FAILURE

	Acutely abnormal	Marked	Mild to marked
Activation of RAAS			
BNP levels (variable)	Usually >100 pg/mL	Usually 800-1200 pg/mL	Usually 200-500 pg/mL
Acute ischemia	Common	Occasional	Rare
Hypertensive crisis	Common	Occasional	Rare
Reparable lesions*	Common	Occasional	Occasional

Abbreviations: BNP, B-type natriuretic peptide; LV, left ventricle; RAAS, renin-angiotensin-aldosterone system.

* Coronary thrombosis, acute mitral regurgitation, etc.

Modified from: Leier CV. Unstable heart failure. In: Colucci WS, Braunwald E, eds. *Atlas of Heart Diseases. Heart Failure: Cardiac Function and Dysfunction.* Vol IV. Philadelphia, Pa: Current Medicine; 1995:9.1-9.14.

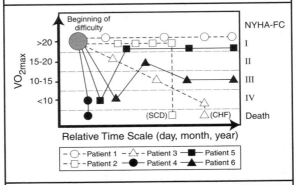

FIGURE 1.1 — TIMELINE OF HEART FAILURE

Abbreviations: CHF, congestive heart failure; NYHA-FC, New York Heart Association functional class; SCD, sudden cardiac death; VO_{2max}, peak oxygen consumption.

As shown in this figure, patients with heart failure present in a variety of ways and have many different long-term event courses. Individuals can remain asymptomatic for long periods of time or have an SCD episode. Others slowly move downhill, with substantive deterioration and symptoms. Many patients initially become quite ill with CHF, but can be treated effectively, with improvement in exercise performance and symptoms.

Modified from: *ACCSAP—Adult Clinical Cardiology Self Assessment Program* (book on CD-ROM). Bethesda, Md: American College of Cardiology; 2000. Based on: Lewis RP, ed. *ACCSAP—Adult Clinical Cardiology Self Assessment Program*. Bethesda, Md: American College of Cardiology; 1999.

crease from 1971. It is likely that there will soon be over a million hospital admissions this year for decompensated CHF. Fifty percent of HF patients are >65 years of age, with the prevalence of the syndrome increasing from 3 per 1000 males aged 50 to 59 years to 27 per 1000 males aged 80 to 89 years.

With the aging US population, HF prevalence will likely be about six million by 2030. The lifetime risk

TABLE 1.3 — COMMON HEMODYNAMIC PATTERNS IN LOW CARDIAC OUTPUT STATES

Pattern	CO	RAP	PAP	PCWP	SVR	SVO₂
Acute pulmonary edema	Variable	↑	Variable	Variable	Variable	Variable
Cardiogenic shock	↓	↑	↑→	↑↑	↑↑	↓↓
Decompensated heart failure	↓	↑	↑↑	↑↑	↑	↓
Acute right ventricular failure	↓	↑↑	→↓	→↓	↑	↓
Massive pulmonary embolism	↓	↑	↑	↑→	↑	↓
Acute aortic/mitral valve insufficiency	↓	↑	↑	↑↑	↑	↓
Cardiac tamponade	↓	↑*	↑*	↑*	↑	↓
Hypovolemic shock	↓	↓	↓	↓	↑	↓

Key: ↑, increased; →, normal; ↓, decreased; ↑↑, markedly increased

Abbreviations: CO, cardiac output; PAP, pulmonary artery pressure; PCWP, pulmonary capillary wedge pressure; RAP, right atrial pressure; SVO₂, mixed venous oxygen saturation; SVR, systemic vascular resistance.

* Equalization of diastolic (RV, PA, LV, and PCWP) pressures is characteristic.

TABLE 1.4 — THE SCOPE OF THE HEART FAILURE PROBLEM

- Lifetime risk of developing congestive heart failure (CHF) is one in five for men and women
- More than four million Americans have symptomatic heart failure (HF)
- 15 million patients affected worldwide
- 700,000 hospital discharges in 1990 with primary diagnosis of HF (fourfold increase from 1971)
- 280,000 deaths in 1990 primarily due to HF
- 50% of HF patients are >65 years old (prevalence of syndrome increases from 3/1000 males aged 50 to 59 to 27/1000 males 80 to 89 years old)
- With aging US population, HF prevalence estimated to be almost six million by 2030
- Mortality overall in symptomatic males is 50% at 24 months in Framingham cohorts
- CHF is the US Health Care Financing Administration largest and most expensive diagnosis-related group
- Each HF hospitalization costs $6,000 to $12,000
- Three-month readmission rates for HF can be 20% to 30%

(age adjusted) for developing CHF is one in five for both men and women based on Framingham data.[167] **Figure 1.2** depicts this dramatic epidemic. HF mortality in symptomatic males was 50% at 24 months in early studies of Framingham cohorts, with 5-year mortality rates noted to be 70% if CHF was diagnosed in a man between 1950 and 1969 and 59% in the era of 1990 to 1999.[167] Furthermore, CHF is the US Health Care Financing Administration's largest and most expensive diagnosis-related group. The high incidence of CHF in the aged (**Figure 1.3**) suggests that our health care system will be severely taxed unless new strategies can be developed and implemented to prevent a baby-boomer HF epidemic.

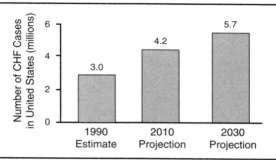

FIGURE 1.2 — PREVALENCE OF CONGESTIVE HEART FAILURE TO DOUBLE BY YEAR 2030 AS US POPULATION AGES*

The number of congestive heart failure (CHF) patients will almost double between the years 1990 and 2030, from three million cases of overt CHF to about six million. Many believe this is a gross underrepresentation of the heart failure problem in the United States.

* According to the American Heart Association (AHA) heart and stroke facts.

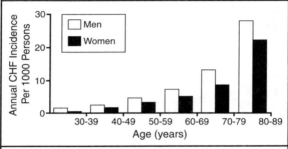

FIGURE 1.3 — INCIDENCE RATES OF CONGESTIVE HEART FAILURE IN FRAMINGHAM HEART STUDY SUBJECTS BY GENDER AND AGE

The annual congestive heart failure (CHF) incidence per 1000 persons is plotted for both men and women, demonstrating a profound and dramatic rise as age increases.

McKee PA, et al. *N Engl J Med.* 1971;285:1441-1446.

2 Etiology

Introduction

Heart failure (HF) is a syndrome representing the final common pathophysiologic pathway of a wide spectrum of myocardial injuries. These varied insults all produce ventricular systolic and/or diastolic dysfunction with resulting systemic circulatory impairment. The myocyte and interstitial matrix injury prompts compensatory processes to maintain homeostasis. The initial workload increase foisted on normal myocytes leads to a variety of molecular biodynamic responses that ultimately cause ventricular remodeling. The pathophysiology of HF is reviewed in more detail in Chapter 3, *Pathophysiology*. However, a multitude of diseases, some better characterized than others, cause cardiac injury, which subsequently leads to HF and reactive congestive states.

Some individuals are uniquely susceptible to specific diseases. Heritable disorders produce molecular alterations that cause cardiac contractile protein production abnormalities. For example, patients with muscular dystrophy often have an associated cardiomyopathy. Patients with myotonic dystrophy and Duchenne's muscular dystrophy frequently die of arrhythmias or congestive heart failure (CHF) (cardiomyopathy) rather than from complications of skeletal muscle weakness. Studies of several kindreds with familial cardiomyopathy have documented a genetic basis for clinically "idiopathic" cardiomyopathy affecting multiple family members. Importantly, clinically healthy members of affected families should undergo serial evaluation, as these inherited disorders may become clinically evident in later life.[76]

Patients with hypertrophic cardiomyopathy have heritable disorders of troponin protein production that lead to obstructive and nonobstructive ventricular hypertrophy and subsequent systolic and diastolic cardiac dysfunction. Cardiac volume or pressure overload states may result from valvular disease or hypertension. By increasing wall stress with ventricular volume or pressure increase, myocyte protein production attempts to bolster the cellular contractile elements in order to meet the increased workloads demanded by these conditions.

Myocyte protein production in these circumstances becomes more representative of fetal than adult patterns. This results in cardiac remodeling and produces contractile and relaxation abnormalities, which ultimately limit systemic perfusion with the metabolic disturbances characteristic of the HF syndrome. Conditions such as myocardial infarction (MI), lymphocytic myocarditis, and ethanol or anthracycline toxicity attack the myocyte itself by inducing apoptosis (premature cell death). Anoxia from acute coronary thrombosis triggers much more rapid myocyte demise by abruptly precipitating cell membrane lysis with subsequent rapid cellular destruction.

Specific Causes of Heart Failure

Table 2.1 lists specific diseases that clinicians should consider when faced with a new HF patient. This organization of HF etiologies was accepted by the World Health Organization (WHO) and International Society and Federation of Cardiology Task Force on the definition of cardiomyopathies in 1996 and summarizes the latest thinking regarding grouping of disease characteristics. The classification scheme is far more complicated than prior schemes that largely focused on dilated, hypertrophic, and restrictive cardiomyopathy. Although these general categories are

TABLE 2.1 — CLASSIFICATION OF HEART FAILURE ETIOLOGIES

Dilated Cardiomyopathy
• Idiopathic

Hypertrophic Cardiomyopathy
• Idiopathic hypertrophic subaortic stenosis
• Hypertrophic obstructive cardiomyopathy
• Hypertrophic nonobstructive cardiomyopathy

Restrictive Cardiomyopathy
• Specific infiltrating diseases
• Idiopathic

Arrhythmogenic Right Ventricular Cardiomyopathy
• Idiopathic right ventricular outflow tract tachycardia
• Arrhythmogenic right ventricular dysplasia

Unclassifiable Cardiomyopathies
• Atypical presentation:
  – Fibroelastosis
  – Systolic dysfunction without dilation
  – Mitochondrial cardiomyopathy
• Mixed presentation (dilated/hypertrophic/restrictive):
  – Amyloidosis (see *Metabolic* section)
  – Hypertension (see *Specific* section)

Specific Cardiomyopathies
• Ischemic
• Valvular obstruction/insufficiency
• Hypertensive
• Inflammatory:
  – Myocarditis:
    › Lymphocytic
    › Giant cell
    › Autoimmune
• Infectious:
  – Chagas' disease
  – Human immunodeficiency virus (HIV)
  – Enterovirus
  – Adenovirus
• Cytomegalovirus
• Bacterial and fungal endocarditis

Continued

Metabolic
- Endocrine:
  - Thyrotoxicosis
  - Hypothyroidism
  - Adrenal cortical insufficiency
  - Pheochromocytoma
  - Acromegaly
  - Diabetes mellitus
- Familial storage disease/infiltration:
  - Hemochromatosis
  - Glycogen storage disease
  - Hurler's syndrome
  - Refsum's disease
  - Niemann-Pick disease
  - Hand-Schuler-Christian disease
  - Fabry-Anderson disease
  - Morquio-Ullrich disease
- Electrolyte deficiency syndromes:
  - Potassium metabolism disturbances (hypokalemia)
  - Magnesium deficiency
- Nutritional disorders :
  - Kwashiorkor
  - Anemia
    › Beriberi
    › Selenium deficiency
    › Nonspecific malabsorption or starvation
- Amyloid (primary, secondary, familial, hereditary, senile)
- Familial Mediterranean fever

General System Disease
- Connective tissue disorders:
  - Systemic lupus erythematosus
  - Polyarteritis nodosa
  - Rheumatoid arthritis
  - Scleroderma
  - Dermatomyositis
- Nonspecific infiltrations and granulomas:
  - Sarcoidosis
- Leukemia

Continued

included in this WHO classification, much more attention is paid to specific disease states causing cardiomyopathies, including the variety of metabolic disturbances and general systemic diseases that can precipitate HF.

Idiopathic dilated cardiomyopathy is diagnosed when no obvious cause of ventricular dysfunction is apparent. Many patients are labeled as having idiopathic dilated cardiomyopathy when CHF or left ventricular dysfunction (LVD) is discovered by happenstance and no other disease can be diagnosed. These patients have normal coronary anatomy, no primary valvular heart disease, no hypertension or diabetes, and no immediately identifiable immunologic or inflammatory process that presaged the discovery of HF.

Hypertrophic cardiomyopathy includes:

- Idiopathic hypertrophic subaortic stenosis (IHSS)
- Hypertrophic obstructive cardiomyopathy (HOCM)

- Hypertrophic nonobstructive cardiomyopathy (HNOCM).

IHSS and HOCM, as well as HNOCM, are distinct entities, genetic in origin, with well-defined heritable characteristics and gene mutations.

Arrhythmogenic right ventricular cardiomyopathy is rare, but it accounts for life-threatening arrhythmias that arise in the right ventricular outflow tract. Fibrotic infiltration of the outflow tract and generalized right ventricular dysplasia account for substantial right-sided CHF in many patients. However, malignant ventricular arrhythmias generally dominate the clinical picture.

Several cardiomyopathies have been lumped into the unclassifiable category. These include cardiomyopathies associated with a variety of presentations that are atypical for CHF, such as:

- Fibroelastosis
- Isolated systolic LVD without chamber dilation
- Mitochondrial cardiomyopathy.

These cardiomyopathies generally do not have profound left ventricular dilation or hypertrophy. They can have restrictive diastolic elements, however. Mixed-presentation cardiomyopathies include hypertensive heart disease and amyloidosis (also included in metabolic cardiomyopathies) because they can present as ventricular dilation, severe hypertrophy, or severe restrictive diastolic dysfunction.

Specific cardiomyopathies include:

- Ischemic heart disease
- Valvular obstruction and insufficiency
- Hypertensive heart disease with HF
- A variety of inflammatory cardiomyopathies that can be difficult to diagnose including:
  - Acute lymphocytic myocarditis
  - Giant cell or autoimmune inflammatory states

– Infectious inflammatory cardiomyopathies such as those seen with Chagas' disease, human immunodeficiency virus, enterovirus, adenovirus, cytomegalovirus, and bacterial or fungal endocarditis.

Important metabolic abnormalities associated with cardiomyopathy include a wide spectrum of endocrinopathies (thyrotoxicosis, hyperthyroidism, Addison's disease, pheochromocytoma, acromegaly, and diabetes). Rare familial storage diseases and infiltrative cardiomyopathies are easily diagnosed by endomyocardial biopsy. These include hemochromatosis and the variety of glycogen storage diseases, such as Hurler's syndrome. Electrolyte deficiency syndromes, either caused by endogenous disease states or exogenous administration of medications, can cause cardiomyopathy. Profound chronic hypokalemia and hypomagnesemia are etiologies of HF. Nutritional disorders, such as kwashiorkor and anemias caused by beriberi (vitamin B_6 deficiency), selenium deficiency, or nonspecific malabsorption or starvation syndromes, can be important to consider, particularly in regions where nutritional compromise is common. Amyloidosis can cause a variety of cardiomyopathies presenting as systolic or diastolic dysfunction. This abnormal proteinaceous myocardial infiltration may be primary, secondary, familial, hereditary, or senile in origin.

General systemic illnesses also precipitate HF and include the large grouping of connective tissue disorders, such as:

- Systemic lupus erythematosus
- Polyarteritis nodosa
- Rheumatoid arthritis
- Scleroderma
- Dermatomyositis
- Sarcoidosis
- Nonspecific granulomatous infiltrations.

As mentioned earlier, systemic muscular dystrophies, in particular, Duchenne's, Becker's, and myotonic dystrophies, are associated with cardiomyopathy. Toxic injury to the heart can result from alcohol, anthracyclines, and irradiation, as well as states in which endogenous catecholamines are elevated. Exogenous administration of catecholamines can also be associated with cardiomyopathy. Peripartum cardiomyopathy represents a heterogeneous group of problems that have been difficult to characterize, including inflammatory autoimmune states and hypertensive heart disease associated with toxemia of pregnancy.

This suggested classification scheme is grouped mainly into cardiomyopathies having certain anatomic characteristics (such as dilated, hypertrophic, and restrictive elements) or cardiomyopathies resulting from a specific injury (ie, ischemic heart disease). It is important to consider the broad etiologic spectrum of HF because many diseases that result in cardiomyopathy can be successfully treated with resolution of the HF syndrome, for example, thyrotoxicosis and myxedema.

The WHO scheme also suggests that cardiomyopathies should be labeled by causal factors as well as by anatomic and physiologic correlates. For example, a patient with prior MI, active ischemic heart disease, and HF associated with congestion and a dilated left ventricle would be most correctly characterized as having a dilated ischemic cardiomyopathy. It should be obvious, as well, that many different diseases can contribute to HF in any given patient. It is not unusual to have combinations of ischemic heart disease and valvular heart disease. Sometimes, the valvular heart disease is precipitated by the ischemic process, such as when an inferolateral-wall MI produces mitral regurgitation. Diagnostic challenges are obvious.

As **Table 2.2** demonstrates, acute HF can be more precisely characterized with respect to etiologies. Acute coronary syndromes, with ischemic ventricular

TABLE 2.2 — PRINCIPAL CAUSES OF ACUTE HEART FAILURE

- Acute coronary syndrome:
  - Acute myocardial infarction
  - Unstable angina pectoris
- Complications of myocardial infarction:
  - Acute mitral regurgitation (papillary muscle rupture or dysfunction)
  - Ventricular septum rupture
  - Cardiac free wall rupture with pericardial tamponade or pseudoaneurysm formation
- Acute valvular catastrophe (sudden mitral or aortic insufficiency):
  - Infective endocarditis
  - Retrograde dissection of aorta (complications of aortic aneurysm)
  - Rupture of myxomatous chorda tendinae
  - Severe and poorly controlled hypertension
- Hypertension (accelerated, malignant, or crises)
- Acute myocarditis
- Sustained atrial or ventricular cardiac arrhythmias (particularly those with rapid ventricular response)
- Acute pulmonary embolism
- Development of peripheral arteriovenous fistulae
- Cardiac tamponade from pericardial effusion of any etiology
- Decompensation of chronic heart failure

dysfunction, MI, or unstable angina, can precipitate profound pulmonary edema. Considering complications of acute MI is particularly important when evaluating the acutely congested patient. Acute mitral regurgitation from papillary muscle rupture or dysfunction, ventricular septal rupture, and cardiac free wall rupture with pericardial tamponade or pseudoaneurysm formation all must be recognized quickly in order to institute lifesaving treatment. Other causes of acute HF include acute myocarditis, sustained atrial or ventricular cardiac arrhythmias (particularly with rapid ven-

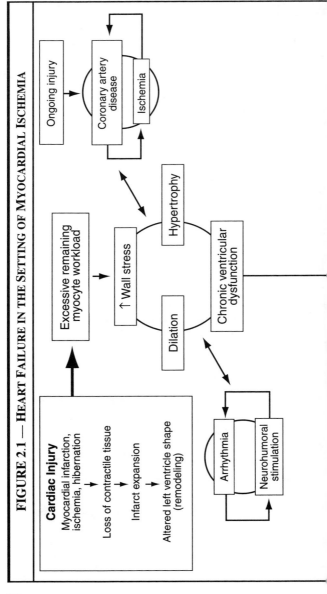

FIGURE 2.1 — HEART FAILURE IN THE SETTING OF MYOCARDIAL ISCHEMIA

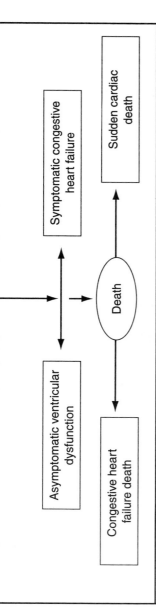

Asymptomatic ventricular dysfunction

Symptomatic congestive heart failure

Death

Congestive heart failure death

Sudden cardiac death

How a specific injury, such as myocardial infarction, precipitates heart failure: Infarction of tissue produces loss of contractile mass, and the subsequent infarct expansion contributes to a remodeled or altered left ventricular shape. Remaining and viable myocytes, though possibly injured by ischemia, have workloads shifted to them, increasing wall stress and further contributing to ventricular dilation and hypertrophy. Dysfunction of the system can produce arrhythmias or neurohormonal perturbation, which will worsen the remodeling process.

Modified from: Pfeffer MA. Cardiac remodeling and its prevention. In: Colucci WS, Baunwald E, eds. *Atlas of Heart Diseases. Heart Failure: Cardiac Function and Dysfunction.* Vol IV. Philadelphia, Pa: Current Medicine; 1995:5.1-5.13.

tricular responses), development of peripheral arteriovenous fistula, cardiac tamponade, and acute pulmonary embolism. Finally, any patient with chronic but stable HF can suddenly deteriorate, with acute decompensation manifest as cardiogenic shock or sudden pulmonary edema when an intercurrent event such as an acute ischemic syndrome or malignant hypertension occurs.

Figure 2.1 demonstrates how one specific disease, coronary artery disease resulting in an acute MI, produces HF. The cardiac injury results from infarction, ischemia, and hibernation, with loss of absolute or functional contractile tissue; infarct expansion follows because of ongoing fibrotic responses that alter ventricular shape. This finally induces ventricular remodeling, both acute and chronic.

The remaining viable myocytes after acute MI have workload shifted to them with increasing wall stress, which further contributes to ventricular dilation and cellular hypertrophy. Mechanical dysfunction of the cardiovascular system can produce arrhythmias or neurohormonal changes that further promote detrimental remodeling. Ultimately, a chronic state of HF develops with patients having asymptomatic ventricular dysfunction or symptomatic CHF. Death may be sudden (usually arrhythmogenic) or may follow a prolonged course in a chronic congestive or low-output state.

3   Pathophysiology

Introduction

Heart failure (HF) is a multifaceted syndrome (**Figure 3**.1). Injury to the heart and the subsequent myocardial reparative processes produce molecular responses, cellular activities, and ultimately anatomic changes. Contraction and relaxation abnormalities develop, with systemic flow decrements that trigger subsequent physiologic responses. This process includes a variety of clinical manifestations ranging from asymptomatic ventricular dysfunction (both systolic and diastolic) to congestive states (volume overload from fluid retention), low cardiac output syndromes, or frank cardiogenic shock. Understanding the negative feedback cycles of HF is critical to unraveling the physiologic responses to cardiac injury.

Molecular Basis of Heart Failure

Heart failure occurs at both the macroscopic circulatory and microscopic molecular biodynamic levels. **Table 3**.1 lists the elements of cardiac contraction that produce cardiac systole and diastole. Cardiac sarcomeres are the central contractile elements of the myocyte. They contain two types of myofilaments that shorten during systole and relax during diastole. The actin and myosin filaments contain proteins, troponin, and tropomyosin, which form cross-bridges when intracellular calcium concentration rises. Calcium-troponin C binding alters the configuration of the adjacent tropomyosin molecule. This exposes the myosin-specific binding site on the actin chain, allowing the myosin head to couple with the actin. As the angle of

41

FIGURE 3.1 — THE FACETS OF HEART FAILURE: COMPLEXITY OF THE SYNDROME

Injury/Induction

- Heritable (familial dilated cardiomyopathy)
- Toxins (ethyl alcohol; anthracyclines)
- Volume overload (aortic insufficiency, mitral regurgitation)
- Pressure overload (hypertension)
- Architectural (patent ductus arteriosis, ventricular septal defect)
- Ischemia (acute myocardial infarction)
- Metabolic (thyrotoxicosis)
- Arrhythmia (supraventricular tachycardia)

Clinical Manifestations

- Asymptomatic ventricular dysfunction
- Congestive state
- Low-output state
- Cardiogenic shock
- Combinations

Physiologic Responses

- Sympathetic nervous system up-regulation
- Renin-angiotensin-aldosterone release
- Inflammation (interleukin [IL]-1, IL-6, tumor necrosis factor alpha [TNFα])

Molecular Biodynamics

- Altered cellular protein/organelle repair-replacement protocols
- Reversions to fetal phenotype
- Accelerated/enhanced protein synthesis
- Apoptosis triggered

Circulatory Changes

- Baroreceptor dysfunction
- Systemic flow decrement
- Autoregulatory system failure (nitric oxide, prostacyclin, endothelin)

Cellular Responses

- Adrenoreceptor abnormalities
- Abnormal receptor coupling/signal
- Abnormal calcium channel fluxes
- Disturbed energetics

Cardiac Dysfunction

- Systolic/contraction abnormalities
- Diastolic/relaxation abnormalities

Anatomic/Morphologic ("Remodeling")

- Myocyte hypertrophy
- Chamber dilation
- Interstitial changes
- Sphericity changes

The heart failure syndrome is complex. Cardiac injury of many sorts has clinical manifestations only after a variety of responses are triggered.

TABLE 3.1 — THE ELEMENTS OF CARDIAC CONTRACTION: REGULATORS OF EXCITATION-CONTRACTION AND REPOLARIZATION-RELAXATION

Myocyte
- Cell membrane:
  - Receptors
  - Channels
- Cell organelles:
  - Nucleus
  - Mitochondria
  - Sarcolemma
  - Sarcoplasmic reticulum
- Cytoplasmic matrix:
  - Regulatory complexes
  - Myofilaments

Cardiac Interstitium
- Arterial/capillary/venous network:
  - Coronary vascular endothelium
- Lymphatic network
- Adrenergic nerve endings:
  - Sympathetic
  - Parasympathetic
- Conduction system
- Basement membrane
- Collagen matrix
- Fibrous tissue
- Fibroblasts
- Macrophages

interaction changes, force is generated. Then the couplet disengages, with the process repeated at new downstream actin sites. The actin and myosin interaction could be described as a rowing motion of actin-myosin interaction. Much of the activity is stimulated by ions passing through a variety of cell membrane channels. The nucleus, the mitochondria, the sarcolemma, and the sarcoplasmic reticulum are responsible for processing signals delivered to the myocyte membrane that coordinate activity in response to physiologic events.

Calcium is essential for the actin-myosin cross-bridges to form. Because the number of cross-bridges accounts for the power of contraction, cardiac contractility depends directly on the concentration of free intracellular myocyte calcium ions. Energy required for cross-bridge formation is supplied by the reduction of adenosine triphosphate to inorganic phosphate and adenosine diphosphate by an enzyme localized in the myosin head. High concentrations of adenosine triphosphate are provided by the exceptionally high density of mitochondria in myocytes where adenosine triphosphate is produced by oxidative phosphorylation. This obligatory oxygen-dependent process depends on adequate coronary blood flow with its rich oxygen supply. In distinction to skeletal muscles, cardiac myocytes are virtually incapable of anaerobic respiration. The release of calcium occurs from cisternal stores when electrical potentials cross the cell membrane. This is a complex and intricately regulated activity. Diastole is also an energy-dependent activity and accounts for approximately one third of all energy-store utilization during the complete cardiac cycle.

The cardiac interstitium (extra myocyte matrix) plays a critical role in excitation contraction and repolarization relaxation characterizing the normal cardiac cycle. The interstitium (extra myocyte matrix) contains the arterial, capillary, and venous blood networks critical to providing adequate energy supply and removing waste products of cellular respiration. The interstitium also contains the lymphatic network of the heart, as well as sympathetic and parasympathetic adrenergic nerve endings and the cardiac conduction system. The collagen and fibrous tissue of the cardiac interstitium is where fibroblasts and macrophages normally can be found, and to a large extent, this zone accounts for the relative stiffness of the heart.

Chapter 2, *Etiology*, discusses the causes of HF. On the other hand, **Table 3**.2 demonstrates how specific and distinct disease processes create the HF milieu through different routes of myocardial injury. Duchenne's muscular dystrophy, for example, is a heritable disorder of nucleolar DNA production. The inability to produce normal contractile elements causes HF. Pressure-volume overload creates a signaling process that results in reversion to the fetal contractile protein phenotype. Myocardial infarction (MI), anthracycline toxicity, and alcoholic cardiomyopathy induce myocyte necrosis and apoptosis with loss of myocytes and contractile mass.

Table 3.3 summarizes the factors important in cardiac remodeling and HF. Myocyte receptor sites that can lead to myocardial hypertrophy range from sites effected by hormones (eg, growth hormone, arginine vasopressin, and angiotensin II) to activation of inflammatory receptors by tumor necrosis factor and a variety of interleukins.

Figure 3.2 shows signaling receptor density changes in HF. It has been demonstrated that failing myocytes have far fewer β_1-adrenergic receptors than nonfailing myocytes. β_2-receptor concentration is, basically, unchanged. The α_1 receptors are seen in more dense fashion in failing hearts while angiotensin II receptors are somewhat decreased. These issues relate to the benefits seen with a variety of agents, including β-blockers and angiotensin receptor blockers (ARBs). It has been argued that complete adrenergic blockade with an agent blocking β_1-, β_2-, and α-adrenergic membrane receptors might be more advantageous than β-blockers having selective β_1 adrenergic blocking capabilities. The recently published COMET study compared outcomes in 3029 subjects with chronic HF, New York Heart Association functional class (NYHA-

TABLE 3.2 — THE HEART FAILURE MILIEU: DIFFERENT ROUTES OF MYOCARDIAL INJURY		
Site	**Mechanism**	**Example**
Nucleolar DNA	Heritable disorder	Muscular dystrophy
Contractile proteins	Perturbation in contractile protein production	Volume overload (mitral regurgitation, aortic insufficiency) Pressure overload (hypertension, aortic stenosis)
Myocardial cell	Necrosis and apoptosis	Myocardial infarct Anthracycline toxicity Alcoholic cardiomyopathy

**TABLE 3.3 — MYOCYTE CELL
MEMBRANE STIMULATORS IMPORTANT IN
HEART FAILURE REMODELING
AND THAT LEAD TO HYPERTROPHY**

- Growth hormone
- Angiotensin II
- Norepinephrine/epinephrine
- Tumor necrosis factor
- Interleukin-1, -5, and -6
- Tissue-derived growth factors
- Endothelium-derived growth factors
- Platelet-derived growth factors
- Arginine vasopressin
- Nitric oxide
- Atrial natriuretic peptide
- Myocyte "stretch"

FC) II to IV with left ventricular (LV) ejection fraction <35%, randomized to treatment with carvedilol vs metoprolol tartrate. At 5 years, all-cause mortality was 5.7% lower in the carvedilol-treated group, suggesting an advantage to the nonselective agent as compared with a selective β_1 blocker. It has been argued, however, that carvedilol should have been compared with the extended release form of metoprolol (metoprolol succinate) and at higher dose targets (200 mg, the metoprolol succinate target in the MERIT-HF trial, vs 50 mg, the metoprolol tartrate target in COMET). Nonetheless, the hypothesis tested in COMET is interesting and important.

Table 3.4 summarizes the differences between myocyte necrosis from acute MI vs apoptosis. Myocyte necrosis is characterized by cellular edema with mitochondrial swelling and membrane integrity loss. There is random DNA degradation and evidence of an inflammatory healing response. Apoptosis, on the other hand, is characterized by cellular involution or shrinking without mitochondrial swelling and, initially, in-

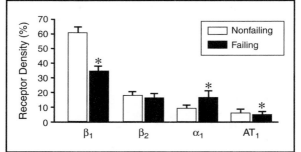

FIGURE 3.2 — ADRENERGIC AND ANGIOTENSIN II RECEPTOR DENSITIES

* $P < 0.05$ vs nonfailing.

This figure shows beta-1 (β_1) and beta-2 (β_2)-adrenergic and angiotensin I (AT_1) receptor densities in nonfailing and failing human left ventricular membrane. Failing myocytes have fewer β_1 receptors than nonfailing myocytes. β_2 receptor density is similar in both failing and nonfailing hearts. Alpha-1 (α_1) receptors are more dense while AT_1 receptors are somewhat decreased in failing hearts. β-Adrenergic blocking drugs that have some β_1 selectivity may be more effective in heart failure.

Bristow MR, et al. *Circ Res.* 1986;59:297-309.

tact organelle and myocyte membranes. Degradation of DNA is organized (multiples of 180 base pair units) rather than random, and there is little accompanying inflammatory response.

Anatomic remodeling in response to molecular injury includes myocyte hypertrophy, cardiac chamber dilation, interstitial fibrosis, and a change in the sphericity index of the ventricle. Shape changes range from globular dilated hearts in individuals with systolic left ventricular dysfunction (LVD) to small obliterated cavities in individuals with hypertrophic cardiomyopathy. **Figure 3.3** summarizes responses to different types of hemodynamic overload that activates myocyte

48

TABLE 3.4 — MYOCYTE NECROSIS VS APOPTOSIS: CHARACTERISTICS

- Necrosis:
  - Cellular edema
  - Mitochondrial swelling
  - Membrane integrity lost
  - Random DNA degradation
  - Inflammatory healing response
- Apoptosis:
  - Cellular involution (shrinkage)
  - No mitochondrial swelling
  - Membranes intact initially
  - Organized degradation of DNA (multiples of 180 base pair units)
  - Little inflammatory response

cellular membrane stretch receptors. Volume overload increases diastolic wall stress, with subsequent cardiac chamber enlargement or eccentric hypertrophy.

Pressure overload increases parallel formation of sarcomeres, which results in concentric hypertrophy. Myocardial mass is significantly increased in both conditions; however, the mass to LV radius is different because of the ventricular chamber dilation seen in eccentric hypertrophy. Whether parallel sarcomere proliferation or series sarcomere proliferation develops probably is related to the interplay of mechanical and intracellular receptor signaling in the different hemodynamic overload states.

Neurohumoral Regulation in Heart Failure

Figure 3.4 graphically presents how neurohumoral regulation of blood flow occurs. A variety of neurohumoral factors control blood flow. The relationship of vascular pressure receptors to the central nervous system, kidney, and adrenal gland triggers

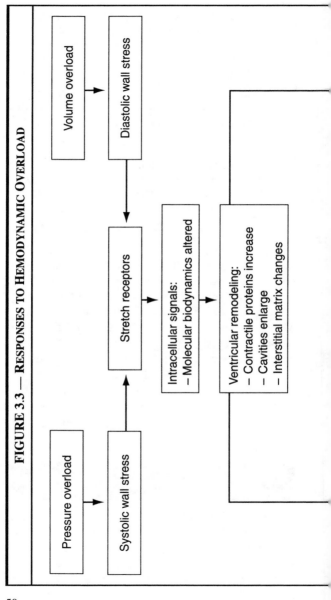

FIGURE 3.3 — RESPONSES TO HEMODYNAMIC OVERLOAD

Volume overload → Diastolic wall stress

Pressure overload → Systolic wall stress

Diastolic wall stress → Stretch receptors ← Systolic wall stress

Stretch receptors → Intracellular signals:
– Molecular biodynamics altered

Intracellular signals → Ventricular remodeling:
– Contractile proteins increase
– Cavities enlarge
– Interstitial matrix changes

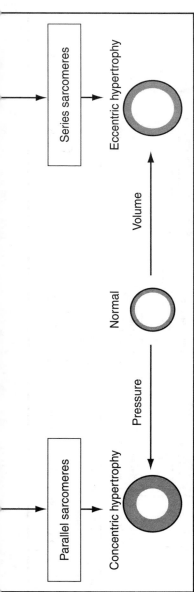

Parallel sarcomeres

Concentric hypertrophy

Pressure

Normal

Volume

Series sarcomeres

Eccentric hypertrophy

Different forms of myocyte loading will induce varieties of hypertrophy. Pressure overload, for example, is more likely to cause concentric hypertrophy, while volume overload stimulates ventricular dilatation wire, so-called eccentric hypertrophy. Whether a parallel sarcomere proliferation or series sarcomere proliferation develops probably is related to the interplay of mechanical and intracellular receptor signaling.

Modified from: Thaik CM, Colucci WS. Molecular and cellular events in myocardial hypertrophy and failure. In: Colucci WS, Baunwald E, eds. *Atlas of Heart Diseases. Heart Failure: Cardiac Function and Dysfunction*. Vol IV. Philadelphia, Pa: Current Medicine; 1995:4.1-4.14.

3

FIGURE 3.4 — NEUROHUMORAL REGULATION OF BLOOD FLOW

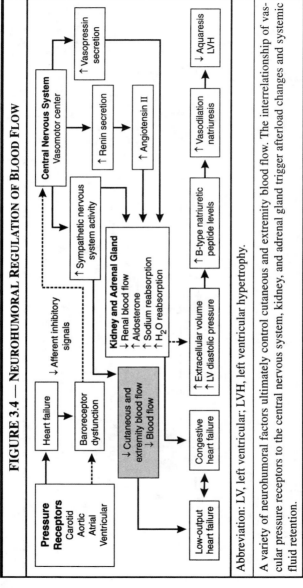

Abbreviation: LV, left ventricular; LVH, left ventricular hypertrophy.

A variety of neurohumoral factors ultimately control cutaneous and extremity blood flow. The interrelationship of vascular pressure receptors to the central nervous system, kidney, and adrenal gland trigger afterload changes and systemic fluid retention.

afterload changes (increased systemic impedance to LV ejection) as well as renal solute and fluid retention. Cutaneous and extremity blood flow decreases in low-output HF. Congestion develops, reflecting renal sodium and water retention and its deposition in organ and systemic interstitial tissues. In addition to sympathetic and parasympathetic nervous system activity, as **Figure 3**.5 demonstrates, a variety of vasoconstricting and vasodilating humors are locally released as flow and vascular wall tension changes to assist with autoregulation of blood movement to peripheral organs. In addition to sympathetic efferent nervous system activity, humoral factors such as epinephrine, angiotensin II, and vasopressin are released when vasodilation occurs. Vasodilators such as endothelium-derived relaxing factor (nitric oxide [NO]), kinins, and prostaglandins also respond to tonic changes in the vasculature.

The neurohumoral regulation and autoregulation of blood flow couples to intrinsic myocardial contractility such that cardiac output is finely tuned and systemic demands can be reasonably met. **Figure 3**.6 summarizes the essence of cardiac output regulation: myocardial preload, afterload, and contractility. Preload is the pressure found in the ventricles at end diastole. Afterload is the systemic vascular resistance against which the ventricles must eject their contents. Contractility is reflected by the inherent cardiac inotropic properties. These three factors are essential for proper stroke volume regulation. Heart rate also determines forward flow, and diminution of stroke volume can result in an increased heart rate to maintain normal forward flow. Arterial pressure is modulated by cardiac and aortic pressure receptors as well as by systemic vascular network autoregulation. The central nervous system controls a variety of medullary, vasomotor, and cardiac control centers with sympathetic and parasympathetic nervous system signaling net-

FIGURE 3.5 — AUTOREGULATION OF BLOOD FLOW

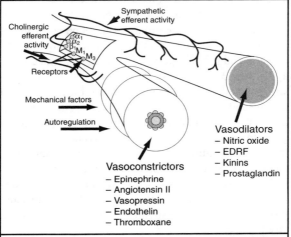

Abbreviations: EDRF, endothelium-derived relaxing factor; M, muscarinic receptors.

A variety of vasoconstrictors and vasodilators respond to local factors and facilitate autoregulation of blood flow to peripheral organs. In addition to sympathetic efferent nervous system activity, humoral factors such as epinephrine, angiotensin II, and vasopressin are released when vasodilation occurs. Vasodilators such as EDRF also respond to tonic changes in the vasculature.

Modified from: Cusco JA, Creager MA. Neurohumoral, renal, and vascular adjustments in heart failure. In: Colucci WS, Baunwald E, eds. *Atlas of Heart Diseases. Heart Failure: Cardiac Function and Dysfunction.* Vol IV. Philadelphia, Pa: Current Medicine; 1995:6.1-6.20.

works activated or inhibited. One can readily see why the introduction of drugs with β-adrenergic blocking or vasodilating properties is challenging.

In HF, as a consequence of altered circulatory dynamics, a variety of neurohormones and inflammatory mediators are generated. **Figure 3.7** presents data from

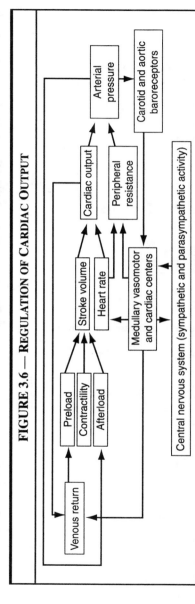

FIGURE 3.6 — REGULATION OF CARDIAC OUTPUT

Cardiac output is primarily regulated by myocardial preload, contractility, and afterload. These three factors are essential for stroke volume to develop adequately. Heart rate ultimately controls forward flow. Arterial pressure is modulated by carotid and aortic pressure receptors, with the central nervous system controlling various aspects of the medullary vasomotor and cardiac centers.

Modified from: Starling MR. Myocardial mechanisms and neurohumoral regulation of the circulation. In: Colucci WS, Baunwald E, eds. *Atlas of Heart Diseases. Heart Failure: Cardiac Function and Dysfunction.* Vol IV. Philadelphia, Pa: Current Medicine; 1995:2.1-2.26

FIGURE 3.7 — NEUROHORMONES AND EJECTION FRACTION

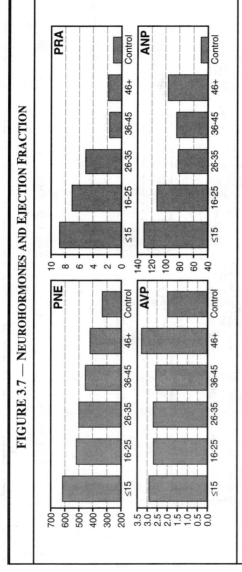

Abbreviations: ANP, atrial natriuretic peptide; AVP, arginine vasopressin; PNE, plasma norepinephrine; PRA, plasma renin activity; SOLVD, Studies of Left Ventricular Dysfunction.

Relationship of neurohormones to ejection fraction SOLVD registry substudy ($n = 895$).

Francis GS, et al. *Circulation.* 1990;82:1724-1729.

the SOLVD trial indicating that as ejection fraction deteriorates, plasma norepinephrine, plasma renin, arginine vasopressin (antidiuretic hormone), and atrial natriuretic peptide levels increase.[37,91,155,276-278,320] **Table 3.5** and **Figure 3.8** summarize the adverse effects of neurohumoral activation in HF. As **Figure 3.8** demonstrates, angiotensin I is converted to angiotensin II by angiotensin-converting enzyme (ACE), mostly in the lung. ACE is, however, found in systemic tissues and in the heart. Other proteases (such as chymase) can also convert angiotensin I to angiotensin II in organs and tissues; therefore, ACE inhibitor (ACEI) use will not block production of all angiotensin II. Thus the interest in use of both ACEIs and ARBs in HF.

As noted in **Table 3.5**, angiotensin II, among other agents, is a potent vasoconstrictor. Angiotensin II enhances sodium reabsorption in the proximal kidney tubule and stimulates adrenal aldosterone synthesis and release. Aldosterone enhances sodium reabsorption along with potassium secretion in the collecting ducts of the kidney. This hormone also seems linked to LV fibrosis and remodeling. Arginine vasopressin (or antidiuretic hormone), another hormone activated by ventricular insufficiency, is a vasoconstricting agent that increases water reabsorption in the medullary collecting duct of the kidney and increases sodium chloride reabsorption in the medullary ascending limb of Henle's loop.

The neurohumoral responses to HF are mediated through the vascular system and the kidney (**Figure 3.9**). The end result of neurohumoral activation includes increased systemic vascular resistance and increased extracellular fluid volume. Elevations in both left and right ventricular filling pressure reflect the combined effects of cardiac dysfunction and neurohormonal response, and the elevated filling pressures in turn provide the stimulus for natriuretic peptide secretion. The elucidation of the natriuretic peptide system[30] and its response to elevated cardiac filling pressures represents a major ad-

TABLE 3.5 — RENAL EFFECTS OF NEUROHUMORAL ACTIVATION IN HEART FAILURE

Vasoconstrictor Activities
- Angiotensin II:
  - Efferent greater than afferent arteriolar constriction
  - Enhanced sodium reabsorption in proximal tubule
  - Stimulates adrenal aldosterone synthesis and release
- Aldosterone:
  - Enhanced sodium reabsorption, with potassium secretion in collecting ducts
- Arginine vasopressin:
  - Increased water reabsorption in medullary collecting duct
  - Increased sodium chloride reabsorption in medullary ascending limb of Henle's loop

Vasodilatory Activities
- Natriuretic peptides:
  - Increase glomerular filtration rate
  - Promote diminished sodium reabsorption in collecting ducts
  - Suppress renin activity
  - Inhibit aldosterone synthesis and release
  - Inhibit vasopressin release
  - Reduce preload and afterload
- Renal prostaglandins:
  - Promote renal vasodilation
  - Decrease tubular sodium reabsorption in ascending limb of Henle's loop
  - Inhibit vasopressin action in collecting ducts

vance in cardiovascular medicine. **Table 3.6** lists the natriuretic peptides and some of their basic properties. B-Type natriuretic peptide (BNP) increases glomerular filtration rate and acts as an endogenous vasodilator by affecting NO release. Because BNP secretion occurs in response to vasoconstriction and salt and water retention, the effects of BNP are not sufficient to overcome the pathophysiology of HF. However, in HF, BNP

FIGURE 3.8 — SYSTEMIC AND TISSUE RENIN-ANGIOTENSIN SYSTEM

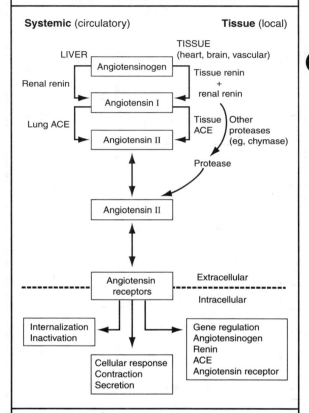

In addition to the conversion of angiotensin I to angiotensin II by angiotensin-converting enzyme (ACE) (found mostly in the lung), "tissue" ACE can be noted in the heart. Other proteases, such as chymase, can account for this buildup of angiotensin II, independent of ACE.

Modified from: Thaik CM, Colucci WS. Molecular and cellular events in myocardial hypertrophy and failure. In: Colucci WS, Baunwald E, eds. *Atlas of Heart Diseases. Heart Failure: Cardiac Function and Dysfunction.* Vol IV. Philadelphia, Pa: Current Medicine; 1995:4.1-4.14.

FIGURE 3.9 — RENAL CONSIDERATIONS IN HEART FAILURE

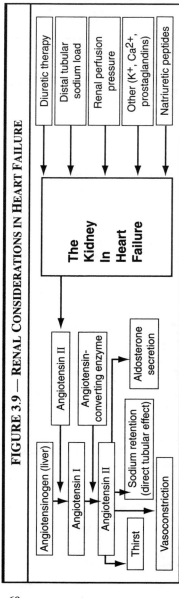

With heart failure, the kidney causes a variety of difficulties based upon the volume presented to it. Renin release is induced by diuretic therapy, diminished tubular sodium load, and decreased renal perfusion pressure. Atrial natriuretic factor and vasopressin can inhibit the release of renin. Renin release stimulates the conversion of angiotensin to angiotensin I, which is then converted by angiotensin-converting enzyme to angiotensin II, causing vasoconstriction, aldosterone secretion, and sodium retention.

Modified from: Cusco JA, Creager MA. Neurohumoral, renal, and vascular adjustments in heart failure. In: Colucci WS, Baunwald E, eds. *Atlas of Heart Diseases. Heart Failure: Cardiac Function and Dysfunction.* Vol IV. Philadelphia, Pa: Current Medicine; 1995:6.1-6.20.

TABLE 3.6 — THE NATRIURETIC PEPTIDES

Acronym	Term	Primary Source
ANP	A-type natriuretic peptide; atrial natriuretic peptide	Cardiac arria
BNP	B-type natriuretic peptide; brain natriuretic peptide	Cardiac ventricles
hBNP	Human B-type natriuretic peptide	Cardiac ventricles
CNP	C-type natriuretic peptide	Endothelium
DNP	Dendroaspic natriuretic natriuretic peptide	Green mamba snake venom

Adapted from: Mills RM, et al. *Congest Heart Fail.* 2002; 8:271.

appears to be the most physiologically important natriuretic peptide. It is a beneficial counter regulatory hormone in HF. The clinical measurement of BNP levels has won rapid acceptance as a useful index of the degree of neurohormonal activation in HF patients.

The prostaglandins, another counterregulatory group of peptides, have an important role in modulating the pathophysiology of HF. These potent compounds, produced in the kidney, promote renal vasodilation. Prostaglandins also decrease tubular sodium reabsorption in the ascending limb of Henle's loop and inhibit the action of vasopressin in collecting ducts. **Figures 3.8** and **3.9** relates these effects to other important factors to consider in HF, including diuretic therapies and electrolyte and solute concentrations. Ultimately, all of these effects result in the potential for congestion and renal dysfunction when HF occurs.

Inflammation and Heart Failure

Recently, cytokines and their role in the development of HF have attracted great attention. These molecules are important elements of any healing process. The heart and circulatory system respond to injury with cytokine activation in a fashion similar to other organs. Up-regulation of proinflammatory and down-regulation of anti-inflammatory cytokines is commonly seen in HF. Tumor necrosis factor can, for example, cause LVD (it is a negative inotropic agent), and it induces myocyte hypertrophy and cardiac chamber dilation. **Figure 3**.10 summarizes data from patients with varying degrees of HF participating in the SOLVD trial. In the upper panel, plasma tumor necrosis factor alpha (TNFα) levels in normal patients are compared with those having NYHA-FC I through IV HF. Patients with more severe HF had higher levels of this cytokine. Furthermore, the data demonstrate an adverse impact on survival in groups having higher TNFα levels (lower panel, **Figure 3**.10).

Pathophysiologically, HF is best characterized by detrimental remodeling. **Table 3**.7 summarizes why remodeling, characterized by myocyte hypertrophy, interstitial matrix stiffening, and chamber enlargement, is deleterious. Although remodeling occurs to compensate for circulatory failure, myocardial hypertrophy results in increased wall stress with disturbed cell energetics as the myocardial oxygen supply:demand ratio is altered unfavorably. With reversion to the fetal cardiac phenotype in compensatory hypertrophy, the myocardial cell contracts less forcefully, resulting in ventricular systolic dysfunction. As the interstitial matrix of the heart adds and alters normal collagenous structure, the ventricles stiffen and diastolic dysfunction shifts the pressure/volume curve upward. Finally, terminally differentiated myocytes induce apoptosis,

FIGURE 3.10 — TUMOR NECROSIS FACTOR IN HEART FAILURE

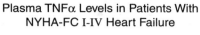

Plasma TNFα Levels in Patients With NYHA-FC I-IV Heart Failure

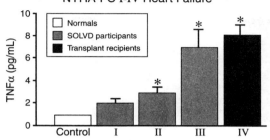

Effect of Plasma TNFα on Survival in SOLVD

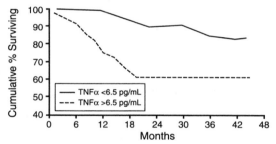

Abbreviations: NYHA-FC, New York Heart Association functional class; SOLVD, Studies of Left Ventricular Dysfunction; TNFα, tumor necrosis factor alpha.

* <0.05 vs control.

In the SOLVD trial, TNFα concentration rose as heart failure worsened *(top)* and was associated with a higher mortality *(bottom)*. Inflammatory cytokines are likely important in both the pathogens of heart failure and as prognostication markers.

Torre-Amione G, et al. *J Am Coll Cardiol.* 1996;27:1201-1206.

TABLE 3.7 — WHY MYOCARDIAL REMODELING IN HEART FAILURE IS DELETERIOUS: REASONS FOR EXACERBATING CARDIAC DYSFUNCTION

Results of Hypertrophy
- Increased wall stress:
  - Disturbed cell energetics (myocardial oxygen supply:demand)

Results of Return to Fetal Myocyte Phenotype
- Myocytes contract with less power:
  - Systolic dysfunction

Results of Abnormal Interstitial Matrix
- Heart stiffens:
  - Diastolic dysfunction

"Growth" Stimuli of Terminally Differentiated Cell
- Apoptosis:
  - Premature senescence or cell death
    › Loss of contractile cell units

causing premature senescence or cell death and, ultimately, further loss of essential contractile units.

By emphasizing individuals at risk for HF and those with asymptomatic LVD, the new joint American College of Cardiology/American Heart Association (ACC/AHA) classification of HF highlights many of the issues outlined in this chapter. **Figure 3.11** presents the new classification. This classification extends, rather than replaces, the time-honored NYHA classification by recognizing risk factors for HF and the long asymptomatic phase of the process.

FIGURE 3.11 — ACC/AHA GUIDELINES: HEART FAILURE DIAGNOSIS AND MANAGEMENT

Structural heart disease → *Symptoms of HF develop* → *Refractory symptoms of HF at rest*

Stage A
(high risk for HF but without structural heart disease or symptoms of HF)

Patients with:
- Hypertension
- Diabetes mellitus
- Family history of CM
- Patients using cardiotoxins

THERAPY
- Smoking cessation
- Treat metabolic disorders
- Exercise
- Limit alcohol, avoid illicit drugs
- ACEI, ARB, ASA in appropriate patients

Stage B
(structural heart disease but without symptoms of HF)

Patients with:
- Previous MI
- LVH
- Asymptomatic LV dysfunction
- Asymptomatic valvular disease

THERAPY
- All stage A measures
- β-Blockers in appropriate patients

Stage C
(structural heart disease with prior or current symptoms of HF)

Patients with:
- Known structural heart disease
- Shortness of breath, fatigue, reduced exercise tolerance, edema

THERAPY
- All stage A measures
- Drugs indicated:
  – ACEI
  – ARB
  – β-Blocker
  – Aldo antag ± digitalis
  – Diuretics
- Na^+/H_2O restriction

Stage D
(refractory HF requiring specialized interventions)

Patients who have symptoms at rest despite maximal medical therapy (eg, those who are recurrently hospitalized or cannot be safely discharged from hospital without specialized interventions)

THERAPY
- Stage A, B, & C measures
- Mechanical assist devices
- Heart transplant
- Continuous IV inotrope palliation
- Hospice care

Abbreviations: ACC/AHA, American College of Cardiology/American Heart Association; ACEI, angiotensin-converting enzyme inhibitor; aldo antag, aldosterone antagonist; ARB, angiotensin receptor blocker; ASA, acetylsalicylic acid; CM, congestive myocardiopathy; HF, heart failure; H_2O, water; IV, intravenous; LV, left ventricular; LVH, LV hypertrophy; MI, myocardial infarction; Na^+, sodium.

Modified from: Hunt SA, et al. *J Am Coll Cardiol.* 2001;38:2101-2113.

3

65

4 Diagnosis

Introduction

The diagnosis of heart failure (HF) no longer rests exclusively on signs and symptoms. Advanced imaging, noninvasive estimates of hemodynamic status, and rapid assessment of neuroendocrine activation now complement the history and physical examination. However, a careful and complete clinical evaluation is still required.[312,316] **Figure 4.1** provides an overview of the important elements of assessing patients for HF. A detailed history can give insight into the functional status of pulmonary, cardiac, gastrointestinal (GI), and neuropsychiatric systems. Physical examination should focus on the heart, lungs, GI tract, integument, and neurologic systems. Subtle but important historic facts and physical examination findings can give insight into the diagnosis of HF, its etiology, precipitating factors, severity, and prognosis. Basic laboratory tests, evaluation of neuroendocrine status with B-type natriuretic peptide (BNP) levels, and noninvasive or invasive assessment of cardiac anatomy and function are also important. Two-dimensional (2-D) and Doppler echocardiographic examinations, BNP levels, and basic laboratory data guide accurate staging of HF and the choice of treatment strategy.

The results of a HF evaluation should provide answers to several critical questions. These are summarized in **Table 4.1**. Does the patient actually suffer from HF and what caused the initial myocardial injury? What precipitated the patient's deterioration? The evaluation must stage the degree of disability. This will allow determination of the patient's short- and long-term prognosis, and it also dictates therapeutic strategies.

FIGURE 4.1 — ASSESSMENT OF HEART FAILURE

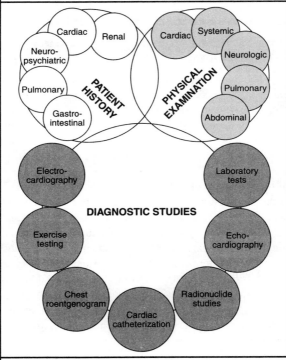

Assessment of heart failure should include a history of the function of the pulmonary, cardiac, gastrointestinal, renal, and neuropsychiatric systems. Likewise, physical examination should focus on the heart, lungs, gastrointestinal tract, integument, and neurologic systems. A variety of studies, including basic laboratory tests and noninvasive or invasive assessment of cardiac function, are important.

Modified from: *ACCSAP—Adult Clinical Cardiology Self Assessment Program* [book on CD-ROM]. Bethesda, Md: American College of Cardiology; 2000. Based on: Lewis RP, ed. *ACCSAP—Adult Clinical Cardiology Self Assessment Program.* Bethesda, Md: American College of Cardiology; 1999:102.

**TABLE 4.1 — INTEGRATION OF
DIAGNOSTIC EVALUATION**

*In the end, results of the heart failure (HF) evaluation
need to be critically assessed so that the following ques-
tions can be answered:*
- Does the patient actually suffer from HF?
- What is the etiology of the syndrome?
- What precipitated the patient's deterioration?
- How severe is the HF syndrome?
- What is the patient's short- and long-term prognosis?
- Is the patient on potentially detrimental medications?
- How should the patient be treated acutely?
- How should the patient be treated chronically?
- Can the disease process be favorably modified? Can
  the HF be controlled?
- What social factors and social support mechanisms
  should be considered as adjunctive measures?

Clinical History

The new American College of Cardiology/Ameri-
can Heart Association (ACC/AHA) classification of
HF (**Figure 3.11**) emphasizes the preclinical phase of
the syndrome. HF represents a "final common path"
for many different forms of heart disease. Forestall-
ing the onset of overt symptoms by vigorous management of patients at risk offers far greater benefit than
more complex interventions for established decompensation. Once symptomatic HF begins, many seemingly
disparate elements of a patient's history might influence diagnosis and management (**Table 4.2**). Generally, HF diagnostic algorithms focus on symptomatic
patients with stable and, usually, reasonably compensated congestive heart failure (CHF) not requiring hospitalization. Complaints that could possibly be related
to CHF include:
- Paroxysmal nocturnal dyspnea
- Orthopnea

TABLE 4.2 — THE CLINICAL HISTORY IN HEART FAILURE: SPECIFIC ISSUES TO EXPLORE

Cardiovascular
- Angina pectoris
- Nonspecific chest pain syndromes
- Fatigue
- Weakness
- Orthostatic faintness
- Palpitations
- Rheumatic disease
- Congenital disease

Pulmonary
- Dyspnea on exertion
- Orthopnea
- Paroxysmal nocturnal dyspnea
- Periodic respirations
- Nocturnal apnea
- Snoring
- Pleurisy
- Cough
- Hemoptysis
- Wheezing

Gastroenterologic
- Abdominal pain
- Abdominal bloating
- Constipation/diarrhea
- Anorexia
- Nausea
- Vomiting

Neurologic/Neuropsychiatric
- Anxiety or panic
- Depression
- Confusion
- Decreased mental acuity

Continued

Renal
• Nocturia
• Oliguria
Systemic
• Edema
• Petechiae/ecchymosis
• Claudication
• Cellulitis
• Weight gain/loss

- Dyspnea on exertion
- Lower extremity edema
- Decreased exercise tolerance
- Unexplained confusion
- Altered mental status
- Nonspecific fatigue
- GI or abdominal symptoms that might relate to mesenteric congestion (such as nausea, abdominal pain, bloating, and a swollen abdomen or ascites).

Physicians often misdiagnose HF, particularly in younger patients, attributing the pulmonary signs and symptoms to asthma or panic attacks. A simple BNP determination may provide critical data in the evaluation of dyspnea.[177]

HF and sleep-disordered breathing syndromes have a complex interaction and are turning out to be intimately linked. On the one hand, sleep-disordered breathing occurs frequently in the setting of advanced HF; on the other, patients with no evident structural heart disease may develop pulmonary hypertension and overt right HF due to sleep apnea. Snoring, intermittent breathing, morning headache, and uncontrollable daytime sleepiness suggest sleep-disordered breathing, which may be either an indicator or a cause of HF.

Nocturia is one of the earliest signs of volume overload. Systemic signs of HF, including edema and weight gain or, when cachexia begins to develop, weight loss despite edema, give insight into the severity of the syndrome. Finally, it is important to round out a patient's presentation with a complete history of comorbidities, particularly the presence of diabetes, obstructive pulmonary disease, collagen vascular diseases, or atherosclerotic events.

Physical Findings

Table 4.3 summarizes important physical findings in HF. In addition to simply obtaining one blood pressure, multiple measurements with the patient supine, sitting, and standing can be helpful in characterizing orthostatic symptoms.

Other vital signs important to note include heart rate and rhythm. Resting tachycardia and atrial fibrillation are markers for a poor prognosis. Pulse pressure is helpful in characterizing the severity of HF. A proportionate pulse pressure (systolic blood pressure – diastolic blood pressure/systolic pressure) <0.25 is associated with poor outcomes. Respiratory rates should be noted as well as the pattern. Periodic respirations indicate severe HF. Tachypnea with minimal exertion, such as climbing up onto the examination table, is also important. An elevated or depressed body temperature also carries important information. HF patients dramatically deteriorate when systemic infections are present. Hypotension can be associated with low-flow states and a grave prognosis.

The cardiovascular examination should include assessment of volume status, such as:

- Elevated jugular venous pressure
- Positive hepatojugular reflux
- Third heart sound
- Sustained cardiac apical impulse
- Pulmonary rales that do not clear with cough

TABLE 4.3 — PHYSICAL EXAMINATION OF HEART FAILURE PATIENTS: SPECIFIC PHYSICAL FINDINGS TO PURSUE

Vital Signs
- Positional blood pressure
- Pulse rate, rhythm, and pulse pressure
- Respiratory rate and pattern
- Temperature

Cardiovascular
- Neck vein distention
- Abdominal-jugular neck vein reflux
- Cardiomegaly
- Displaced, sustained, or hyperkinetic apical impulse
- Chest wall pulsatile activity (right ventricular lift)
- Gallop rhythms
- Heart murmurs (especially aortic, mitral, tricuspid, and pulmonic insufficiency or stenosis murmurs)
- Diminished S_1 or S_2
- Friction rub
- Peripheral venous insufficiency

Pulmonary
- Rales
- Rhonchi
- Prolonged expiration
- Wheezes
- Dullness to chest percussion
- Friction rubs

Abdominal
- Ascites
- Hepatosplenomegaly
- Pulsatile liver
- Decreased bowel sounds
- Obesity

Neurologic
- Mental status abnormalities

Systemic
- Acrocyanosis
- Edema
- Temporal muscle wasting
- Cachexia

4

- Peripheral edema not caused by simple venous insufficiency.

Heart murmurs are often heard in HF patients. Murmurs of mitral, tricuspid, and pulmonic insufficiency are important, as are those suggesting aortic stenosis or insufficiency. Generally, severely ill HF patients have soft heart sounds. Friction rub in a setting of acute HF suggests infarction or inflammatory pericarditis-myocarditis. Rales and basilar dullness often indicate pulmonary congestion; however, CHF with significant pulmonary hypertension can be present with no pulmonary findings of note on the physical examination.

Inspection and palpation of the abdomen might demonstrate ascites, hepatosplenomegaly, a pulsatile liver, or decreased bowel sounds, all common findings in congested individuals, particularly when significant tricuspid insufficiency develops.

Neurologic and general systemic findings may include mental status abnormalities and evidence of systemic hypoperfusion, including acrocyanosis. Systemic edema may or may not represent a congestive state, but with all of the other physical examination elements it assists one in making the diagnosis.

Finally, the physical examination should include attention to findings that suggest presence of other systemic illnesses.

Natriuretic Peptides in the Diagnosis of Heart Failure

The introduction of a rapid point-of-care assay for BNP into clinical practice represents a significant improvement in the diagnosis and management of HF. As outlined in Chapter 3, *Pathophysiology*, the neurohormonal response to HF results in intravascular volume expansion and, in conjunction with cardiac dysfunction, elevation of ventricular filling pressure. Elevated

74

filling pressure then stimulates pro-BNP secretion and cleavage into the active moiety, BNP, and a biologically inactive fragment, NT-proBNP. (**Table 4**.4 and **Figure 4**.2) Determination of BNP levels provides useful data in several different clinical settings:

- *Emergency department diagnosis.* The BNP Multinational Study[186] included 1586 subjects presenting with acute dyspnea. A BNP level over 100 pg/mL had 96% sensitivity and 76% specificity for the diagnosis of HF vs other causes of dyspnea. Another single center emergency department study randomly assigned 452 acutely dyspneic patients to an evaluation strategy including BNP determination or not with time to discharge and total treatment cost. When BNP levels were known, 75% of patients were hospitalized vs 85% in a well-matched group of patients ($P = 0.008$). Length of hospital stay and total costs were less when BNP levels were known.[200] Like many other clinical tests, BNP levels are most useful when the pretest likelihood of disease is in the midrange.

- *Prognosis.* Elevated BNP levels indicate increased risk for readmission and death due to HF and increased risk for sudden death. Elevated BNP levels in acute coronary syndromes are also predictive of both short- and long-term mortality. A Framingham database study demonstrated that in 3346 persons without diagnosed HF, higher BNP and NT-BNP levels predicted risk of death and cardiovascular events even after adjustment for traditional cardiovascular risk factors and even at levels below those currently used to diagnose HF.[180,303]

- *Management.* Increasing BNP levels during hospitalization indicate a high risk of death or readmission, and a level >500 pg/mL at dis-

TABLE 4.4 — KEY DISTINGUISHING FEATURES OF THE VENTRICULAR NATRIURETIC PEPTIDES		
Characteristic	BNP	NT-proBNP
Components	BNP molecule	NT fragment (1-76 aa) NT-proBNP (1-108 aa)
Molecular weight	3.5 kd	8.5 kd
Hormonally active	Yes	No, inactive peptide
Genesis	Cleavage from NT-proBNP	Release from ventricular myocytes
Half-life	20 minutes	120 minutes
Clearance mechanism	Neutral endopeptidase clearance receptors	Renal clearance
Increases with normal aging	+	++++
Higher in women	+	?
Correlation with estimated glomerular filtration rate	-0.20	-0.60
Approved cutoff(s) for CHF diagnosis	100 pg/mL	Age <75 years: 125 pg/mL Age ≥75 years: 450 pg/mL

Approved for assessment of CHF severity	Yes	No
Approved for prognosis in ACS	Yes	No
Prospective ED studies completed	Yes	No
Community screening studies completed	Yes	Yes
Available at the point of care	Yes	No
Date of entry on US market	November 2000	December 2002

Abbreviations: aa, amino acid; ACS, acute coronary syndrome; BNP, B-type natriuretic peptide; CHF, congestive heart failure; ED, emergency department; NT, N-terminal.

Modified from: McCullough PA, et al. *Rev Cardiovasc Med.* 2003;4:72-80.

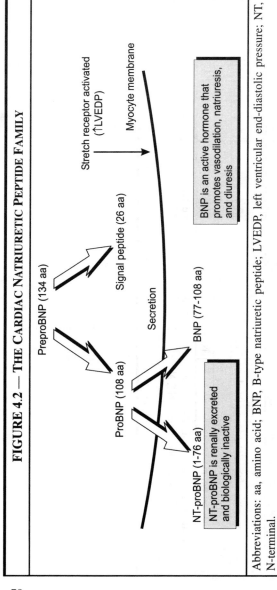

FIGURE 4.2 — THE CARDIAC NATRIURETIC PEPTIDE FAMILY

PreproBNP (134 aa)

Signal peptide (26 aa)

ProBNP (108 aa)

BNP (77-108 aa)

Secretion

Myocyte membrane

Stretch receptor activated (↑LVEDP)

BNP is an active hormone that promotes vasodilation, natriuresis, and diuresis

NT-proBNP (1-76 aa)

NT-proBNP is renally excreted and biologically inactive

Abbreviations: aa, amino acid; BNP, B-type natriuretic peptide; LVEDP, left ventricular end-diastolic pressure; NT, N-terminal.

Modified from: McCullough PA, et al. *Rev Cardiovasc Med.* 2003;4:72-80.

charge also indicates a high risk of death or re-admission within 6 months.

As with any other clinical finding or laboratory data, BNP levels must be integrated into an overall assessment of the patient's condition. BNP assays do not provide complete or infallible information. However, the argument for including BNP levels in a complete admission and discharge database in the management of HF is well-documented and compelling. Furthermore, one needs to remember that age, female gender, and renal dysfunction are associated with higher BNP levels.

Other Laboratory Procedures

Table 4.5 lists laboratory procedures to consider in HF patients. Moderate anemia turns out to be common in patients with long-standing severe HF, and its pathogenesis is not clearly understood. Perhaps it relates to the inflammatory cytokine activation that occurs in this setting. Significant anemia can adversely affect circulatory dynamics, and transfusions or bone marrow–stimulating hormone infusions may be an essential element of therapy. Leukocytosis might point toward infection. Thrombocytopenia can develop with severe hepatosplenomegaly due to right HF. Further insight into hepatic function as it relates to congestion comes from prothrombin times and specific liver function tests. Serum electrolytes, blood urea nitrogen (BUN), and serum creatinine taken as a whole create a more complete picture of metabolic status.

Hyponatremia correlates with severity of neurohumoral activation and degree of congestion. Hypokalemia reflects the effects of diuretics and salt consumption. Hyperkalemia becomes important when aldosterone antagonists, angiotensin receptor blockers (ARBs), or angiotensin-converting enzyme inhibitors (ACEIs) are being administered either alone or, as is

TABLE 4.5 — LABORATORY PROCEDURES TO CONSIDER IN HEART FAILURE PATIENTS

- B-type natriuretic peptide (BNP) levels
- Complete blood count
- Serum electrolytes
- Blood urea nitrogen
- Serum creatinine
- Liver function tests:
  - Serum transaminases
  - Lactic dehydrogenase
  - Alkaline phosphatase
  - Bilirubin (direct and indirect)
  - Albumin
- Hemoglobin A_{1C}
- Prothrombin time
- Lipid levels
- High-sensitivity C-reactive protein (Hs-CRP)
- Thyroid function studies
- Anemia evaluation
- Arterial blood gases
- Urinalysis:
  - Proteinuria
  - Hematuria
  - Pyuria
  - Glycosuria
  - Ketonuria
- Biochemistry screen:
  - Magnesium
  - Uric acid
  - Calcium
- Serum drug levels:
  - Digoxin
  - Phenytoin
  - Quinidine
  - Procainamide

now more frequent, in combination. Metabolic alkalosis with elevated carbon dioxide (CO_2) levels is often coupled to hypokalemia and can create particularly difficult problems when trying to wean an intubated CHF patient from a ventilator. Elevation of BUN and serum creatinine give the clinician some insight into the severity of intrinsic renal disease and relative hypoperfusion. Prerenal azotemia, BUN elevation out of proportion to creatinine level, suggests excessive diuresis.

Hemoglobin A_{1C} measurements help in assessing control of diabetes. Lipid profiles with high-sensitivity C-reactive protein measurements may help in designing atherosclerosis prevention programs. Thyroid function studies are mandatory to exclude occult hyperthyroid and hypothyroid states masked by HF, particularly in patients taking amiodarone. Obtain arterial blood gases if pulmonary embolism is considered. Proteinuria is a significant risk factor for adverse outcomes in patients with atherosclerosis and diabetes. Drug levels may be helpful in assessing drug toxicity.

Not every laboratory test is indicated in every patient with or suspected of having HF. Minimal testing profiles should include:

- Complete blood count
- Complete metabolic profile:
  - Serum electrolytes
  - BUN
  - Serum creatinine
- Biochemistry screen that includes:
  - Uric acid
  - Calcium
  - Phosphorus
  - Magnesium
  - Liver function tests
  - Urinalysis
- BNP level
- Urinalysis.

Imaging Tests

Table 4.6 details the main and most common ancillary diagnostic tests utilized when assessing a patient with HF. They include:

- Chest x-ray
- Electrocardiogram (ECG)
- 2-D and M-mode echocardiogram
- Pulsed Doppler echocardiogram.

These evaluations are often supplemented by first-pass or gated radionuclide ventriculograms, computerized tomographic (CT) cardiac scans, or magnetic resonance imaging (MRI). Many patients will go on to cardiac catheterization with coronary angiography and hemodynamic assessments. Alternatively, a variety of noninvasive cardiac imaging studies are designed to quantitate the degree of ischemic, hibernating, and scarred myocardium: dobutamine stress echocardiography, dipyridamole stress echocardiography, thallium scintigraphic studies, exercise radionuclide scintigraphic studies, and gadolinium MRI. The clinician should design the most appropriate sequence of diagnostic tests based upon each individual's particular clinical presentation and the potential for therapeutic interventions.

■ Chest X-Ray

As **Table 4.6** points out, the cardiothoracic ratio and chamber size estimates can be helpful. Pulmonary vascularity and congestion, pleural effusions, or segmental fissure fluid gives an indication of the severity of the congestion.

■ Electrocardiogram

The ECG confirms heart rate and rhythm, may indicate ventricular hypertrophy, and may indicate coronary heart disease by Q waves. It is important to assess

TABLE 4.6 — COMMON ANCILLARY DIAGNOSTIC TESTS

Chest X-ray
- Cardiothoracic ratio
- Cardiac chamber size and shape
- Pulmonary vascularity and congestion
- Pleural effusion
- Mass lesions or infiltrates
- Mediastinal configuration
- Great-vessel abnormality
- Vascular/cardiac calcifications

Electrocardiography
- Rhythm:
  - Atrioventricular coupling
  - Atrial fibrillation
  - Ventricular arrhythmias
- Heart rate
- Evidence of hypertrophy
- Q waves
- P mitrale/pulmonale
- Interventricular conduction disturbances (QRS duration)
- QRS voltage
- Digitalis effects
- Metabolic ST-T wave changes

Echocardiography (2-D/M-mode)
- Chamber size and shape
- Valve integrity and motion (quantitation of stenosis)
- Fractional shortening of ventricles
- Mean circumferential fiber shortening
- Mitral E point to septal separation
- Systolic wall thickening
- Wall-motion analysis
- Estimation of wall stress
- Exercise and pharmacologic stress (wall motion)
- Tissue characterization
- Pericardial effusion
- Pericardial restriction
- Detection of shunts

Pulsed Doppler Echocardiography
- Quantification of valve stenosis/regurgitation:
  - Estimation of pulmonary artery pressure
  - Estimation of stroke volume and cardiac output
- Determination of diastolic filling characteristics

intraventricular conduction disturbances and QRS duration in light of the benefit of biventricular multisite resynchronization pacing protocols. QRS voltage is also important, because this diminishes dramatically with loss of functional myocardium.

■ Echocardiography

Echocardiography has become the single most important procedure in the evaluation of a patient suspected of having symptomatic HF. M-mode, 2-D, and Doppler studies allow evaluation of cardiac chamber size and shape, valve integrity and motion, degree of valvular stenosis or insufficiency, and assessment of global systolic and diastolic function. Presence or absence of pericardial effusion is best determined by echocardiography. Doppler studies can estimate right ventricular systolic pressure, detect shunt lesions, and characterize abnormal diastolic filling patterns. If required, transesophageal echocardiography provides outstanding images and alleviates some of the problems encountered with transthoracic studies.

■ Other Imaging Techniques

Table 4.7 summarizes noninvasive imaging techniques useful in HF patients and provides a comparison of specific information obtained from each. For example, if a surgical operation such as infarct exclusion or mitral valve repair for mitral regurgitation is planned, CT or MRI studies might be extremely important. MRI defines cardiac anatomy, characterizes tissue patterns, and may be the best method to quantify cardiac mass and chamber dimensions. Gadolinium imaging with MRI studies is valuable in identification of scarred regions of the myocardium. It is, however, expensive.

The major limitation of CT scans of the heart is motion artifact. The major advantage is that cross-sectional views with spatial and density orientation

84

TABLE 4.7 — COMPARISON OF NONINVASIVE IMAGING TECHNIQUES IN HEART FAILURE

Observation	M-Mode EchoC	2D EchoC	Doppler EchoC	Gated RNVG	First-Pass RNVG	MRI	CT
Anatomic relationships	+++	++++	+	+	+	++++	+++
Tissue characterization	+++	+++	++	0	0	+++	+++
Wall motion	++	++++	+	++	++++	+++	+++
Hypertrophy	++++	++++	0	0	0	+++	+++
Wall thickening	++++	++++	0	0	0	+++	++
Valvular pathology	++	++++	++++	0	0	++	+++
Valvular regurgitation and stenosis	++	++++	++++	0	0	+++	++
Hemodynamics	+	+	++++	0	0	0	0
Diastolic function	++	+++	++++	0	++	+++	+++
Stress exercise	0	++++	0	++++	++++	+	0
Pharmacologic stress	0	++++	0	++++	++++	++	0
Lower cost/easy availability	++++	++++	+++	++	++	+	+

Abbreviations: CT, computed tomography; EchoC, echocardiography; MRI, magnetic resonance imaging; RNVG, radionulide ventriculography.

Key: 0 - ++++, Relative Utility Scale.

appear to be better than echocardiographic or radionuclide studies. CT scans also provide precise images of great-vessel orientation, as does MRI. New CT techniques quantify coronary artery calcification. Whether this is useful is yet to be proved. Both gated and radionuclide first-pass ventriculography are standard techniques for determining systolic ventricular function. Coupling myocardial perfusion studies to radionuclide ventriculography can more precisely characterize ischemic cardiomyopathies.

Assessment of Functional Capacity

Quantifying exercise limitation is important in evaluating patients with HF. A variety of approaches are used. **Figure 4.3** presents several popular protocols. These protocols, used to stage a patient's HF, relate exercise stress to oxygen (O_2) consumption. When choosing a particular protocol, slow upward ramping of stress, as in the Weber-Janicki, modified Naughton, or Balke protocols, is preferable to the rapid onset high stress load of the Bruce protocol. Often, measurement of O_2 consumption and CO_2 production is coupled to the exercise testing protocols (so-called "metabolic" exercise testing) to determine the respiratory exchange ratio (O_2 consumed divided by CO_2 produced at peak exercise). Adequate maximum exercise occurs when the respiratory exchange ratio is greater than 1:10. This indicates that the subject achieved anaerobic threshold, the point at which more CO_2 is produced than O_2 consumed.

If a patient cannot surpass anaerobic threshold and reach a respiratory exchange ratio of >1:10, limitations other than cardiac function are usually present. This should prompt a search for other problems, including pulmonary difficulties, anemia, or other metabolic or peripheral muscle disease. The peak VO_{2max} (ml O_2/kg/min) at maximum exercise is an important prognostic variably (**Figure 4.3**). As **Table 4.8** indicates, there are many noncardiac causes of dyspnea and exercise intolerance. Metabolic exercise testing with gas-exchange analysis will help to clarify these important issues.

Summary

Our goal is to integrate all of the information obtained to precisely characterize patients' clinical circumstances. **Table 4.9** demonstrates how this is done in differentiating systolic from diastolic dysfunction. Diastolic dysfunction occurs in one third to one half of patients with symptomatic CHF. Remember that the clinical features of HF may be similar whether left ventricular (LV) systolic function is normal or depressed. The pathophysiology of HF with normal systolic ventricular function is different, however, from that in patients with depressed LV ejection fraction. Furthermore, the history and physical examination, along with clinical measurements, help to distinguish diastolic from systolic failure. For example, patients with hypertensive heart disease, particularly those with severe LV hypertrophy, often experience HF because of diastolic dysfunction. In **Table 4.9**, the plus signs favor the diagnosis, and the minus signs indicate that the finding tends to exclude the diagnosis. **Table 4.10** describes the New York Heart Association functional classification.

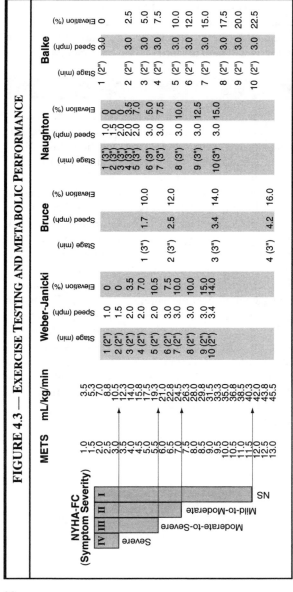

FIGURE 4.3 — EXERCISE TESTING AND METABOLIC PERFORMANCE

Abbreviation: METS, metabolic equivalents (of oxygen consumption); NS, not significant; NYHA-FC, New York Heart Association functional class.

Quantifying exercise limitation is important in many heart failure patients, and a variety of protocols often are used. All attempt to relate certain levels of stress to oxygen consumption and metabolic equivalence. When choosing a particular protocol, clinicians should realize that slow upward ramping of stress, as in the Weber-Janicki; modified Naughton, or Balke protocols for assessment of heart failure, is preferable to the high-stress-load Bruce protocol, which attempts to precipitate ischemic electrographic responses quickly.

Modified from: ACCSAP—Adult Clinical Cardiology Self Assessment Program (book on CD-ROM). Bethesda, Md: American College of Cardiology; 2000. Based on: Lewis RP, ed. ACCSAP—Adult Clinical Cardiology Self Assessment Program. Bethesda, Md: American College of Cardiology; 1999:145.

4

TABLE 4.8 — NONCARDIAC CAUSES OF DYSPNEA AND EXERCISE INTOLERANCE

Cause	Resulting Problems
Anemia	Diminished oxygen-carrying capacity with high cardiac output states
Chest wall deformity	Inadequate ventilation
Malingering	Psychogenic dyspnea syndromes or inadequate effort on exercise
Obesity	Increased workload demands, hyperventilation syndromes, restrictive lung disease
Peripheral vascular disease	Impaired muscle perfusion
Physical deconditioning	Inefficient systemic circulation
Pulmonary Abnormalities	
Airflow limitations (COPD)	Obstructed ventilation
Restrictive alveolar disease	Inadequate ventilation
Ventilation/perfusion	Impaired gas-exchange mismatch

Abbreviation: COPD, chronic obstructive pulmonary disease.

TABLE 4.9 — SYSTOLIC VS DIASTOLIC DYSFUNCTION IN HEART FAILURE: ISSUES TO CONSIDER

Parameters	Systolic	Diastolic
History		
Coronary heart disease	++++	+
Hypertension	++	++++
Diabetes	+++	+
Valvular heart disease	++++	−
Paroxysmal dyspnea	++	+++
Acute presentation	+	+++
Physical Examination		
Cardiomegaly	+++	++
Soft heart sounds	++++	+
S_3 gallop	+++	+
S_4 gallop	+	+++
Hypertension	++	++++
Mitral regurgitation	+++	+
Rales	++	++
Edema	+++	+
Jugular venous distention	+++	++
Chest Roentgenogram		
Cardiomegaly	++	+
Pulmonary congestion	+++	+++
Electrocardiogram		
Low voltage	+++	−
Left ventricular hypertrophy	++	++++
Q waves	+++	+
Echocardiogram		
Low ejection fraction	++++	−
Left ventricular dilation	+++	−
Left ventricular hypertrophy	++	++++

Key: +, favors diagnosis; +, somewhat; ++, moderately; +++, strongly; ++++, very strongly; −, tends to exclude diagnosis.

TABLE 4.10 — NEW YORK HEART ASSOCIATION FUNCTIONAL CLASSIFICATION (NYHA-FC I-IV)

NYHA-FC I
- *No physical activity limitation:* ordinary physical exercise does not cause undue fatigue, chest pain, palpitations, or dyspnea

NYHA-FC II
- *Slight limitation of physical activity:* patient is comfortable at rest, but ordinary activity results in fatigue, chest pain, palpitations, or dyspnea

NYHA-FC III
- *Marked limitation of physical activity:* patient is comfortable at rest, but less than ordinary activity results in fatigue, chest pain, palpitations, or dyspnea

NYHA-FC IV
- *Unable to carry out any physical activity without discomfort:* symptoms of fatigue, chest pain, palpitations, or dyspnea are present even at rest, with increased discomfort with any physical activity

5
Clinical Trials Shaping Heart Failure Therapeutics

Introduction

We are fortunate to have had large numbers of heart failure (HF) patients enrolled in carefully designed and effectively controlled clinical trials with morbidity and mortality end points. These studies have provided objective information that has shaped our practice of evidence-based medicine. Evidence-based medicine relies on clinical trial experience to guide individual patient care. Treatment strategies based on clinical trial results are more likely to improve outcomes. Adherence to these protocols eventually provides one measure of clinical practice quality. Nonetheless, clinical trials cannot answer all important questions and they have some limitations. **Table 5.1** reviews the advantages and disadvantages of clinical trials.

Over the past 2 decades there have been about 100 clinical trials, ranging from several dozen randomized participants to many thousands of patients; these have impacted significantly our practice with regard to HF management. **Table 5.2** and **Table 5.3** summarize clinical trials and registries relevant to HF. Because of the dizzying array of trials and their acronyms, **Table 5.2** groups the trials listed in **Table 5.3** according to subject. The studies are listed in alphabetical order according to the trial acronym in both **Table 5.2** and **Table 5.3**.

Vasodilator Trials

The first large-scale mortality end-point clinical trial in HF was the initial V-HeFT-I.[64] This landmark

TABLE 5.1 — ADVANTAGES AND DISADVANTAGES OF CLINICAL TRIALS

Advantages
- Most precise science
- Best evidence for determining harm/benefit of therapies
- Calculation of impact of interventions
- Clarify specific groups of patients likely to benefit
- Study specific therapeutic/intervention techniques in rigorous fashion

Disadvantages
- Difficult to study the "art of medicine"
- Cannot address all important questions
- Surgical procedures difficult to study
- Inflexible by design
- Long duration (ignore intercurrent developments)
- Difficult to include concurrent advances
- Study populations may not represent real-world practice (ascertainment bias)
- Expensive
- Adequate sample size can be problematic
- Focus largely on questions industry wishes to explore
- Generally designed to study add-on therapies
- Focus on quantitating things that can be counted
- Some things that are important cannot be counted

study of 642 men with moderate congestive heart failure (CHF) was pivotal because vasodilators (hydralazine [HYD] and isosorbide dinitrate [ISDN]) decreased mortality in CHF patients. At the time, this was a controversial hypothesis; attention in HF populations had focused on inotropic drugs. This trial set the stage for interventions with entirely new classes of drugs such as angiotensin-converting enzyme inhibitors (ACEIs) (**Figure 5.1**).

CONSENSUS demonstrated a profound reduction in mortality in severely ill hospitalized CHF patients when enalapril was added to digoxin and diuretics.[74] This study was the first to explore the neurohormonal hypothesis that clinical benefit in HF patients could be achieved by blocking neurohumoral compensatory systems rather than increasing inotropy or decreasing afterload.

V-HeFT-II compared the combination of HYD/ISDN with enalapril, but in patients who were less ill (outpatients) than those studied in CONSENSUS.[66] Enalapril resulted in a greater mortality reduction than did the direct-acting vasodilator combination, although HYD/ISDN improved ejection fraction (EF) more.

At the same time V-HeFT-II was running, additional studies in even less-ill HF patients were ongoing, including the SOLVD program.[37,91,155,276-278,320] This endeavor pitted enalapril against placebo in outpatients with systolic left ventricular dysfunction (LVD) EF <35%. Asymptomatic patients were enrolled in the SOLVD Prevention Trial. Patients with mild to moderate symptomatic CHF (generally, New York Heart Association functional class [NYHA-FC] II/III) were enrolled in the SOLVD Treatment Trial. Baseline medications in the Treatment Trial were diuretics and digoxin, but in the Prevention Trial, enalapril was first-line therapy for asymptomatic systolic LVD. Enalapril significantly reduced mortality and morbidity as well as ischemic events such as acute myocardial infarction (MI) and hospital admissions for unstable angina during long-term follow-up. This observation, coupled with the findings of ACEI post-MI (AIRE, AIREX, CATS, SAVE, SMILE, TRACE[6,118,151,227,289,299]) and with ACEIs as a primary prevention in patients at risk for atherosclerotic events (HOPE), are probably the

TABLE 5.2 — CLINICAL HEART FAILURE TRIALS AND OUR THERAPEUTIC KNOWLEDGE BASE

Angiotensin-Converting Enzyme Inhibitors/Angiotensin Receptor Blockers Post-MI/CHF
- AIRE (ramipril)
- AIREX (ramipril)
- CATS (captopril)
- SAVE (captopril)
- SMILE (zofenopril)
- TRACE (trandolapril)
- VALIANT (valsartan)

Angiotensin-Converting Enzyme Inhibitors in CHF
- APRES (ramipril)
- ATLAS (lisinopril)
- CONSENSUS (enalapril)
- MHFT (captopril)
- OVERTURE (omapatrilat)
- SOLVD (enalapril)
- SPICE Registry
- V-HeFT-II (enalapril)

Angiotensin Receptor Blockers in CHF
- CHARM (candesartan)
- ELITE (losartan)
- ELITE-II (losartan)
- RESOLVD (candesartan)
- RESOLVD: β-Blocker Study (candesartan/metoprolol)
- SPICE (candesartan)
- STRETCH (candesartan)
- V-HeFT (valsartan)

Antiarrhythmics in CHF
- AMIOVERT (amiodarone)
- BASIS (amiodarone)
- CAMIAT (amiodarone)
- CHF-STAT (amiodarone)
- DIAMOND-CHF (dofetilide)
- DIAMOND-MI (dofetilide)
- EMIAT (amiodarone)
- GESICA (amiodarone)
- MUSTT (variable)
- PIAF (diltiazem/amiodarone)
- SWORD (*d*-sotalol)

Automatic Implantable Cardioverter
Defibrillators in CHF
- AMIOVERT
- CABG Patch
- CASH
- COMPANION
- MADIT
- MADIT-II
- MIRACLE
- MIRACLE ICD
- MUSTIC
- SCD-HeFT

β-Blockers in CHF
- BEST (bucindolol)
- CAPRICORN (carvedilol)
- CIBIS (bisoprolol)
- CIBIS-II (bisoprolol)
- COMET (carvedilol)
- COPERNICUS (carvedilol)
- MDC (metoprolol)
- MERIT-HF (metoprolol)
- MEXIS (metoprolol)
- PRECISE (carvedilol)
- MOCHA (carvedilol)

Calcium Channel Blockers in CHF
- MACH-I (mibefradil)
- PRAISE (amlodipine)
- V-HeFT-III (felodipine)

Hypertension and CHF Prevention
- ALLHAT (α-blockers)
- CAPP (captopril)
- HOPE (ramipril)
- MICRO-HOPE (ramipril)

Inotropes in CHF
- DIG (digoxin)
- DIMT (ibopamine)
- Enoximone: Oral Enoximone in Moderate to Moderately Severe CHF (enoximone)
- LIDO (levosimendan)
- OPTIME-CHF (milrinone)

Continued

- PICO (pimobendan)
- PRIME-II (ibopamine)
- PROMISE (milrinone)
- PROVED (digoxin)
- RADIANCE (digoxin)
- VEST (vesnarinone)
- Xamoterol (xamoterol)

Other Treatments in CHF
- ACCLAIM (vasogen immune modulation)
- EPHESUS (eplerenone)
- Growth Hormone: Preliminary Study of Growth Hormone in the Treatment of Dilated Cardiomyopathy
- HIPPOCRATES
- IMAC (IVIG)
- IMPRESS (omapatrilat)
- RALES (spironolactone)
- RENAISSANCE (etanercept)

Strategies in CHF
- CASS (surgery)
- ELVD (exercise)
- ESCAPE (right-heart catheterization)
- SHOCK (early revascularization)
- SUPPORT (right-heart catheterization)
- WATCH (anticoagulation)

Vasodilators in CHF
- FIRST (prostacyclin)
- Hy-C (hydrazaline)
- MOXCON (moxonidine)
- PROFILE (flosequinan)
- RITZ (tezosentan)
- REFLECT (flosequinan)
- V-HeFT-I (hydralazine/isosorbide dinitrate)
- VMAC (nesiritide)

Abbreviations: CHF, congestive heart failure; IVIG, intravenous immunoglobulin; MI, myocardial infarction.

Note: See Chapter 13, *List of Trial Acronyms* for full trial name definitions and **Table 5.3** for details of study.

most important observations made (further discussion follows).[124-127,172,196,274]

The SOLVD Prevention Trial demonstrated a significant reduction in the combined end point of CHF morbidity (hospitalizations for worsening CHF) and mortality. This landmark event suggested an ACEI (enalapril) could attenuate progression to symptomatic CHF when used as first-line drug treatment in asymptomatic or minimally symptomatic patients with systolic LVD. This observation brought a paradigm shift in the treatment of HF, which now focuses on prevention strategies more than end-stage management.

ACEI are critical post-MI when systolic LVD or symptomatic clinical CHF appears. The SAVE trial with captopril demonstrated improved survival and functional status and reduced repeat MI rates in acute infarction patients with EFs <40%.[227] AIRE,[6] SMILE,[11] and TRACE,[151,289] using ramipril, zofenopril, and trandolapril, have confirmed the SAVE trial observations and suggest that ACEIs begun shortly after MI have significant benefits for patients with either asymptomatic systolic LVD or mild clinical HF. One post-MI study that did not demonstrate a reduction in mortality was CONSENSUS-II, in which enalaprilat was routinely administered intravenously early after MI and then changed to enalapril long-term. Timing and drug-dosing issues in this study likely negated benefits. Several larger trials with ACEIs also confirmed that therapy after MI reduces short-term mortality. The ISIS-4 and the GISSI-3 trials included patients with a wide spectrum of EF and suggested that early administration of captopril or lisinopril translates into postinfarction benefit. Interestingly, omapatrilat, a combination ACEI/neutral endopeptidase inhibitor (designed to block the degradation of natriuretic peptides), also did not prove better than an ACEI (OVERTURE).

The benefits of digoxin in patients with HF have been debated for over 2 centuries. The DIG trial was

TABLE 5.3 — SELECT CLINICAL TRIALS, REGISTRIES, AND EXPERIENCES HAVING RELEVANCE TO HEART FAILURE

Acronym (Full Title)	Study Design	Findings	Therapeutic Implication
ACCLAIM (Advanced Chronic Heart Failure Clinical Assessment of Immune Modulation Therapy)[292]	Double-blind, randomized study of vasogen immune modulation therapy for CHF morbidity and mortality reduction (n = 1200)	Trial ongoing	Will give insight into nonspecific immune modulation techniques in CHF patients
AIRE (Acute Infarction Ramipril Efficacy)[6]	Effect of ramipril on morbidity and mortality of survivors of AMI with clinical evidence of HF	Significant reduction in mortality noted with ramipril; findings compliment SAVE, SMILE, TRACE, GISSI-III, ISIS-IV	ACEI therapy should be routinely started postinfarct when CHF or LV systolic dysfunction present
AIREX (Acute Infarction Ramipril Efficacy Extension)[118]	Long-term (mean 59 months) follow-up of AIRE study patients	Average duration of "masked" trial drug 12 months but even poststudy difference in mortality was 39% for placebo vs 28% for ramipril groups (RR, 36%; 95% CI, 0.15-0.52; $P = 0.002$)	Ramipril post-MI with HF has large and sustained benefit
ALLHAT (Antihypertensive and Lipid-Lowering Treatment to Prevent Heart Attack Trial)[10,159]	Randomized, double-blind, active drug-controlled clinical trial of chlorthalidone, doxazosin, amlodipine, or lisinopril with composite end point of fatal CAD event or nonfatal MI (prevention of CHF) secondary end point (n = 24,335)	Doxazosin arm discontinued early because the diuretic produced equal mortality to the α-blocker but there were fewer strokes; combined CVD events with the risk of CHF doubled with doxazosin at 4 years (RR, 2.04; 95% CI, 1.79-2.32; $P < 0.001$)	Doxazosin appears inferior to at least a thiazide diuretic for hypertension for the prevention of CVD events, particularly HF (chlorthalidone, amlodipine, and lisinopril arms still running)
AMIOVERT (Amiodarone vs ICD in IDC Mortality Trial)[283]	178 patients with IDC and VT randomized to received amiodarone or ICD	No significant difference in mortality between groups	Small study that did not demonstrate ICD benefit; hypothesis being more intently studied in SCD-HeFT

APRES (Angiotensin-Converting Enzyme Inhibition Post Revascularization Study)[148]	After revascularization, angina patients with EF 0.30 - 0.50 (asymptomatic) were randomized (double-blind) to ramipril or placebo	ACEIs reduced composite end point of cardiac death, AMI, CHF, or recurrent angina (RR, 0.58; 95% CI, 0.07-0.80; $P = 0.031$)	More evidence for benefits of ACEI for broad spectrum of LVD/HF patients
ATLAS (Assessment of Treatment With Lisinopril and Survival)[17,218,259,296]	Survival study of high- (~35 mg) vs low-dose (~5 mg) lisinopril in moderate-to-severe CHF ($n = 3164$)	No mortality benefit with high ACEI dose, but hospitalizations and morbidity diminished	High target ACEI dose likely wise
AVID (Antiarrhythmics vs Implantable Defibrillators)[14,92,201]	Randomized comparison in resuscitated (near fatal VF or symptomatic VT) patients with EF <0.40 of AICD device vs antiarrhythmics (amiodarone or sotalol) ($n = 1016$)	Survival greater in AICD group (75.4% vs 64.1% at 3 years; a 39% ± 20% reduction in mortality)	In survivors of VF or symptomatic VT with low EF, AICDs appeared superior to antiarrhythmic drugs for improving survival
BASIS (Basal Antiarrhythmic Study of Infarct Survival)[43]	Randomized, open clinical trial of antiarrhythmic (amiodarone) therapy in post-MI patients with asymptomatic complex arrhythmias (frequent multiform or repetitive VAs); control group, individualized antiarrhythmic treatment (drug titrated to eliminate arrhythmia), routine low-dose amiodarone (200 mg daily) ($n = 312$)	Probability of survival (combined end point of mortality and sudden death, sustained VT/VF) increased with routine amiodarone prescription (10 group 1 vs 5 group 2 vs 15 control deaths)	Low-dose amiodarone appears to decrease mortality the first year after MI when certain asymptomatic VAs are present; though not an HF trial, mean EF was 0.43 ± 16
BEST (β-Blocker Evaluation of Survival Trial)[31]	Patients receiving standard treatment randomized to placebo or bucindolol to determine a mortality benefit in moderate-to-severe HF	No benefit noted in NYHA-FC III/IV CHF patients with bucindolol	Either bucindolol is a β-blocker not associated with benefit in HF or population studied was resistant to specific drug

Continued

5

Acronym (Full Title)	Study Design	Findings	Therapeutic Implication
BNP (Breathing Not Properly)[186]	Randomized study in emergency department of B-type natriuretic peptide assessment in dyspnea patients with suspected CHF (n = 1586)	50% of patients dyspneic from CHF; BNP >100 pg/mL 74% sensitive, 90% specific, and diagnostic accuracy was 74%	Routine BNP measurement in challenging cases with dyspnea can help to diagnose CHF
CABG Patch (Coronary Artery Bypass Graft Patch)[34,78]	CAD patients undergoing CABG with EF <0.36 and abnormal SAEKG randomized to patch-ICD vs control with mortality primary end point (n = 1055)	At mean follow-up of 32 ± 16 months, the hazard ratio for death was 1.07 (95% CI 0.81-1.42; P = 0.64) (no significant interaction between ICD and baseline variables)	Survival not improved with ICD during CABG in patients with depressed EF and abnormal SAEKG
CAMIAT (Canadian Amiodarone Myocardial Infarction Arrhythmia Trial)[47,48]	Patients (n = 120) 6 to 45 days post-infarction without EF entry criteria but EKG VA followed for combined end point of arrhythmic death or resuscitated VF; all-cause mortality and cardiac mortality secondary end point	Primary end point benefited with amiodarone but toxicity great (42.3% of treatment group stopped amiodarone by 2 years), all-cause mortality not reduced	Though not an HF trial per se, some patients obviously had LVD; amiodarone may benefit select post-MI patients, but difficult to tolerate
CAPPP (Captopril Prevention Project)[122]	Prospective, randomized, open-label trial of captopril vs conventional (diuretics/β-blockers) antihypertensive therapies with composite end point of fatal/nonfatal MI, stroke, other CVD deaths (n = 10,985)	No difference in events was observed (RR, 1.05; 95% CI, 0.90-1.22; P = 0.52)	Captopril and conventional therapy did not differ in hypertensives for CVD end points, but captopril dosing odd and low
CAPRICORN (Carvedilol Post-Infarction Survival Control in Left Ventricular Dysfunction)[50]	Double-blind, placebo-controlled, mortality end point trial of carvedilol added to "best" MI treatment when LVEF <40% and BP >90 mm Hg	All-cause mortality (RR, 0.77; 95% CI, 0.60-0.98; P = 0.031), but combined mortality/hospitalization end point not impacted (RR, 0.92; 95% CI, 0.80-1.07; P = 0.296)	Most recent MI β-blocker study ("modern era"), again suggesting importance of drugs in this setting

Study	Description	Results	Comments
Carvedilol Program: Effect of Carvedilol on Morbidity and Mortality in Patients With Chronic Heart Failure[39,71,85,210]	Combined analysis of four distinct studies with varied patient enrollment criteria and outcome measures analyzing safety data regarding mortality events ($n = 1094$)	Carvedilol reduced mortality from 7.8% to 3.2% ($P < 0.001$); findings also suggested higher doses better	More data supporting use of β-blocker (this one with α-blocking properties as well) in CHF; there may be important differences between selective and nonselective β-blockers in CHF
CASH (Cardiac Arrest Study-Hamburg)[158,201]	Prospective, randomized trial of AICD vs antiarrhythmics (amiodarone, propafenone, metoprolol) in SCD survivors ($n = 349$, 61 with AICD)	With a mean follow-up of 57 ± 34 months, survival was only slightly higher in the AICD group (RR, 0.766; 97.5% CI, 1.112; $P = 0.081$)	This study only suggested AICD therapy slightly better (in nonsignificant sense) in SCD survivals; though not an HF trial, the mean EF was about 45%
CASS (Coronary Artery Surgery Study)[8]	Survival–end point, randomized study of CABG vs "best" medical therapy for ischemic heart disease with 10-year follow-up ($n = 780$) performed over a decade ago	CABG did not prolong life or prevent infarcts compared with medical therapy except when EF <50%	One of several studies to suggest that coronary revascularization is important in patients with HF and ischemia
CAST (Cardiac Arrhythmia Suppression Trial)[51-53,119]	Mortality end point trial of encainide and flecainide post-MI in patients with PVCs and, generally, LVD	Potent NYHA-FC I antiarrhythmic agents increase mortality in MI patients with LVD	Avoid Vaughn-Williams class I antiarrhythmics in CHF if possible
CATS (Captopril and Thrombolysis Study)[299]	Double-blind, placebo-controlled, clinical trial of captopril in patients receiving streptokinase post-MI with remodeling LV function end points ($n = 298$)	Occurrence of LV dilation significantly lower ($P = 0.018$) and development of CHF less ($P = 0.04$) with captopril	Early post-MI remodeling study showing ACEI benefits
CHARM (Candesartan in Heart Failure-Assessment of Reduction in Mortality and Morbidity)[110,187,189,229,286,321]	Three independent, international, parallel, placebo-controlled mortality end point trials of candesartan cilexetil in patients with NYHA-FC II/IV CHF: 1) LVEF ≤40%, ACEI treated ($n = 2300$); 2) LVEF ≤40%, ACEI intolerant ($n = 1700$); 3) LVEF >40%, not treated with ACEI ($n = 2500$)	In baseline adjusted mortality results, 9% decrease ($P = 0.032$) with 21% CHF hospitalization reduction ($P < 0.0001$)	Highly significant reduction in CV deaths and CHF hospitalizations in ACEI-intolerant patients and those taking ACEI. Only CHF hospitalization reduced when EF >40%

5

Continued

Acronym (Full Title)	Study Design	Findings	Therapeutic Implication
CHF-STAT (Congestive Heart Failure–Survival Trial of Antiarrhythmic Therapy)[84,270]	Survival study of amiodarone vs placebo in CHF patients with 10 PVC/h	Amiodarone overall did not improve survival compared with placebo	Did not support hypothesis that amiodarone was generally helpful in CHF
CIBIS (Cardiac Insufficiency Bisoprolol Study)[61,101,160]	Bisoprolol (a selective β-blocker) added to diuretics/vasodilator with mortality end point	Trend toward morbidity reduction without statistically significant reduction in mortality	Added to portfolio suggesting β-blockers beneficial in some CHF patients
CIBIS-II (Cardiac Insufficiency Bisoprolol Study-II)[62]	Placebo-controlled, mortality end point trial of 2647 patients given bisoprolol for 16 months	Significant reduction in mortality	Longer trial than CIBIS-I with more ill population and higher dose of bisoprolol; 34% reduction in mortality, particularly SCD
CIDS (Canadian Implantable Defibrillator Study)[72,201,263]	SCD survivors randomized to either AICD or amiodarone ($n = 659$)	There was a nonsignificant 20% RR reduction (95% CI, 0.07–0.40; $P = 0.142$) in total mortality with a stronger trend toward reduction of arrhythmic death (RR reduction of 33%; 95% CI, 0.07–0.58; $P = 0.094$); the study was stratified for EF <$/$>0.35% with mean EF of 0.33% and 12% with EF <0.20%	Perhaps AICD better than amiodarone for secondary prevention of SCD syndrome
COMET (Carvedilol or Metoprolol European Trial)[21,22,88,108,238,261]	Active drug-control design with metoprolol tartrate compared with carvedilol in 3029 stable CHF patients	Carvedilol was better than shorter-acting metoprolol in reducing mortality	Study gives insight into possible superiority of nonselective, vasodilating β-blocker in mild-to-moderate CHF
CONSENSUS (Cooperative North Scandinavian Enalapril Survival Study)[74]	Enalapril added to digoxin and diuretic in severe HF (NYHA–FC IV)	Dramatic reduction in mortality at 6 months	ACEI an extremely important addition in CHF
COPERNICUS (Carvedilol Prospective Randomized Cumulative Survival)[213]	Carvedilol vs placebo in 2289 NYHA-FC IIB/IV CHF patients with mortality end point	35% reduction in mortality	Most-ill CHF group studied to date with β-blocker

DIAMOND-CHF (Danish Investigations of Arrhythmia and Mortality on Dofetilide–Congestive Heart Failure)[150,290]	Double-blind, placebo-controlled, clinical trial of dofetilide in symptomatic CHF and severe LVD with mortality the primary end point ($n = 1518$)	During a median follow-up of 18 months, there was no difference in mortality (~41%) with the hazard ratio 0.95 (95% CI, 0.81-1.11), but dofetilide decreased CHF hospitalization and converted AF more but with a 3.3% incidence of torsades in the dofetilide group	Dofetilide appears to be a risky drug to use in CHF patients with a long-term neutral effect on mortality but significant proarrhythmia problem
DIAMOND-MI (Danish Investigations of Arrhythmia and Mortality on Dofetilide–Myocardial Infarction)[150,290]	Double-blind, placebo-controlled, mortality end point clinical trial of dofetilide in MI survivors with severe LVD ($n = 1510$)	Morbidity and mortality no different in dofetilide and placebo groups	No antiarrhythmic agent post-MI reduces mortality unlike ACEI and β-blockers
DIG (Digitalis Investigation Group)[84,106,209,284]	Survival evaluation to assess the mortality effect of digoxin vs placebo in stable CHF when used with ACEI and diuretics (n ~7000)	No survival benefit with digoxin but morbidity (CHF hospitalizations) reduced	Digoxin is an important agent in CHF to reduce morbidity but likely has no mortality impact
DIMT (Dutch Ibopamine Multicenter Trial)[300]	Double-blind, digoxin- and placebo-controlled trials of ibopamine in mild-to-moderate CHF with exercise capacity, neurohormonal measurements, and NYHA-FC end points ($n = 161$)	Digoxin increased exercise time after 6 months compared with placebo ($P = 0.008$), whereas ibopamine effective only in patients with EF >0.30%; plasma norepinephrine and renin decreased by both	Digoxin likely clinically beneficial while ibopamine results need to be placed into the perspective of the other prematurely stopped trials showing detriment (eg, PRIME-II)
ELITE (Evaluation of Losartan in the Elderly)[153,231,234]	Tolerability and morbidity/mortality study of 722 patients >65 years of age with NYHA-FC II, III, or IV CHF assigned to either losartan or captopril	Losartan better tolerated and had lower mortality than captopril	The AII receptor blocker losartan may play a role in CHF
ELITE-II (Evaluation of Losartan in the Elderly-II)[93,153,232]	Comparison of losartan to captopril with mortality end point in 3152 NYHA-FC II/IV CHF patients with EF <40% and age >60 years	No mortality difference between ACEI and AII blocker in this trial; however, trial not powered to demonstrate equivalence	Role of AII blockers in CHF still not clear; one should not substitute an AII blocker for an ACEI routinely

5

Continued

105

Acronym (Full Title)	Study Design	Findings	Therapeutic Implication
ELVD (Exercise in Left Ventricular Dysfunction)[107]	Patients post–non-Q MI with EF <0.40 randomized to 6-month exercise training or control groups with LV volumes and function end points ($n = 77$)	Exercise training decreased LV volumes and increased EF	Long-term exercise in post-MI CHF prevents remodeling
EMIAT (European Myocardial Infarction Amiodarone Trial)[142]	Patients 5 to 21 days postinfarction with EF <40% randomized ($n = 1486$) with mortality primary end point	Primary end point, death, not reduced by amiodarone, but combined end point of arrhythmic death/resuscitated cardiac arrest reduced slightly	No definite benefit with amiodarone in post-MI LVD, and toxicity of drug significant in this study
ENABLE-1 and 2 (Endothelin Antagonist Bosentan for Lowering Cardiac Events in Heart Failure)[143,208]	1613 NYHA IIIB/IV CHF patients randomized to placebo or bosentan; mean EF = 25% with 66% ischemics; 1.5 year follow-up	321 patients died or were hospitalized for CHF in placebo vs 312 in bosentan groups ($P = 0.9$)	Bosentan did not improve survival or hospitalization for CHF in patients with severe CHF on usual therapy
Enoximone: Oral Enoximone in Moderate to Moderately Severe CHF[295]	Randomized, placebo-controlled trial of enoximone in combination with digoxin/diuretics with exercise and symptoms primary end points ($n = 102$)	Enoximone did not improve exercise tolerance or symptoms during 16 weeks of therapy with significantly more dropouts (46% vs 25%) and more deaths (10 vs 3; $P <0.05$)	Worse survival and questionable benefits raise serious questions about this PDE inhibitor
EPHESUS (Eplerenone Neurohormonal Efficacy and Survival Study)[233,235]	6632 patients randomized to placebo or eplerenone early post-MI if systolic LVD (EF <40%) and CHF	During mean follow-up of 16 months, there was a significant mortality reduction ($RR = 0.85$; 95% CI, 0.75-0.96; $P = 0.008$)	Adding eplerenone, an aldosterone antagonist, to optimal therapy for patients with post-MI HF reduced mortality
ESCAPE (Evaluation Study of Congestive Heart Failure and Pulmonary Artery Catheterization Effectiveness)[260]	Randomized trial designed to test the long-term safety and efficacy of CHF hospital therapy guided by hemodynamics vs clinical assessment; primary end point is number of days patients are hospitalized or death during 6-month follow-up ($n = 500$)	Trial ongoing	Study adds commentary on "hemodynamically" guided CHF therapy

FACET (Flosequinan ACE Inhibitor Trial)[184]	Exercise and QOL end point trial with flosequinan 100 mg or 75 mg added to digoxin, diuretic, and ACEI	Subsequent mortality trial demonstrated increase in death rates; drug may make patient feel better but at a cost of higher mortality
FIRST (Flolan International Randomized Survival Trial)[49]	Mortality study of conventional therapy vs continuous IV epoprostenol (a prostacyclin) in end-stage CHF	This study was terminated prematurely due to increased mortality and clinical deterioration in the epoprostenol group	Prostacyclin not an option for chronic parenteral infusion in HF; mortality is increased
GESICA (Grupo de Estudio de la Sobrevida en la Insuficiencia Cardiaca en Argentina)[86]	Placebo-controlled study of amiodarone in moderate-to-severe CHF, assessing mortality as a primary end point	Mortality was significantly reduced with amiodarone (42%) compared with placebo (53%)	Suggested amiodarone can be used in some CHF patients
Growth Hormone: Preliminary Study of Growth Hormone in the Treatment of Dilated Cardiomyopathy[94,171]	Open-label, case series of GH given to IDC patients with LVD, QOL, clinical class as end points (n = 6)	All parameters improved during 3-month treatment period, including the development of hypertrophy	Small pilot study suggesting GH may be beneficial but hypertrophy concerning
HOPE (Heart Outcomes Prevention Evaluation)[124-127,172,196,274]	Randomized 2 × 2 factorial design of ramipril and vitamin E in ~9500 patients at high risk for CV events, including development of CHF	Impressive reductions in CV events, including development of CHF, particularly in diabetics with ACEI but not vitamin E	ACEI (ramipril) is a powerful agent when given early to patients at risk of CV events with benefit not entirely due to BP reduction
Hy-C (Hydralazine vs Captopril: Effect on Mortality in Patients With Advanced Heart Failure)[98]	Comparison of captopril or hydralazine tailored to hemodynamic goals with respect to mortality in NYHA-FC III/IV CHF (n = 117)	Captopril survival at 1 year 81% vs hydralazine 51% (P = 0.05)	Early study demonstrating ACEI better than hydralazine/nitrates despite achieving same hemodynamics
IMAC (Intervention in Myocarditis and Acute Cardiomyopathy With IV Immunoglobulin)[190]	Randomized, double-blind, multicenter trial in 61 patients with new-onset cardiomyopathy who received IVIG or placebo	No differences in outcomes, with LVEF being primary end point	IVIG likely plays no role in benefiting patients with new-onset cardiomyopathy presumed to be inflammatory in etiology

5

Continued

Acronym (Full Title)	Study Design	Findings	Therapeutic Implication
IMPRESS (Inhibition of Metalloprotease by BMS-186716 in a Randomized Exercise and Symptoms Study)[255]	Randomized, double-blind, clinical trial with omapatrilat or lisinopril in NYHA-FC II/IV CHF patients with exercise primary end point ($n = 573$)	Exercise tolerance improved similarly in two groups but few CVD events with omapatrilat (7% vs 12%; $P = 0.04$) and trend toward fewer deaths plus CHF admissions (RR, 0.53; 95% CI, 0.28-0.96; $P = 0.035$)	Pilot trial suggesting omapatrilat could have some advantages over ACEI in CHF; angioedema with omapatrilat needs to be resolved
LIDO (Levosimendan Infusion vs Dobutamine [in low output HF])[221]	Randomized, double-blind multicenter comparison of the efficacy and safety of 24-hour levosimendan infusion vs dobutamine in severely decompensated CHF patients ($n = 200$)	Both drugs hemodynamically active with fewer deaths in group exposed to levosimendan at 180-day follow-up (concomitant medications not specified/controlled)	Study raises the important question of long-term effects of short-term vasoactive drug infusion (tachycardia noted and concerning) etiology
MACH-1 (Mortality Assessment in Congestive Heart Failure 1)[166]	Mibefradil, a T-type calcium channel blocker compared with placebo in 2390 patients with NYHA-FC II/III CHF on ACEI, diuretics, digoxin	Mibefradil increased mortality by 11% compared with placebo	Calcium channel blockers remain a concern in CHF, with mibefradil likely adversely interacting with drugs that prolong QT interval
MADIT (Multicenter Automatic Defibrillator Implantation Trial)[198]	Randomized trial of AICD vs conventional therapy in post-MI patients with EF ≤40%, NSVT, and having had sustained VT at EPS	AICD leads to better survival in this high-risk ASCVD population with HF; β-blockers and amiodarone did not appear to have significant impact on hazard ratio	Provided an alternative strategy for treatment of select patients with HF and life-threatening VAs
MADIT-II (Multicenter Automatic Defibrillator Implantation Trial-II)[199]	Routine ICD implants (without EPS) in patients with EF ≤30% and prior MI; (2:1 randomization) ($n = 1232$)	Marked reduction (trial stopped early) in death (hazard ratio = 0.69; 95% CI, 0.51-0.93; $P = 0.016$) with slight increase in CHF hospitalizations	ICD insertion should be considered in all post-MI patients with reduced LVEF
MDC (Metoprolol in Dilated Cardiomyopathy)[301]	Effect of metoprolol vs placebo on survival in dilated cardiomyopathy	Compared with placebo, metoprolol patients had improved symptoms and cardiac function; 34% fewer primary end points of death or transplant listing with metoprolol	Provided some support for β-blocker use in CHF patients, but study design (end points) criticized

MERIT-HF (Metoprolol CR/XL Randomized Intervention Trial in Heart Failure)[129,191]	Tested efficacy of adding the β-blocker long-acting metoprolol to standard therapy in NYHA-FC II/IV CHF ($n = 3991$), morbidity and mortality end points	Highly significant (35%) decrease in mortality with long-acting metoprolol; trial stopped early	Additional evidence supporting β-blocker use in mild-to-moderate CHF; long-acting metoprolol properties different from carvedilol and bisoprolol
MEXIS (Metoprolol and Xamoterol in Ischemic Syndromes)[226]	Double-blind, active drug-controlled evaluation of β-blockers (one with significant ISA activity) in MI patients with HF; exercise, QOL, and symptoms primary end points ($n = 210$)	Generally little difference between drugs, but mortality 4.7% at 1 year for metoprolol and 5.8% for xamoterol with more withdrawals from xamoterol (22% vs 17%)	Findings are concerning when juxtaposed to adverse events noted in the xamoterol HF trial
MHFT (Munich Mild Heart Failure Trial)[149]	NYHA-FC II CHF patients randomized to captopril 25 mg bid vs placebo with progression of HF major end point ($n = 170$)	Fewer patients progressed to NYHA-FC IV in the captopril group (11% vs 26%; $P = 0.01$)	Early study suggesting ACEI benefit even at low dose
MICRO-HOPE (Microalbuminuria, Cardiovascular, and Renal Outcomes–HOPE substudy)[125]	Substudy of HOPE trial assessing development of nephropathy in diabetics ($n = 3577$)	In diabetics, ramipril lowered CV events by 25% (95% CI, 0.12-0.36; $P = 0.0004$) and over nephropathy by 24% (95% CI, 0.12-0.36; $P = 0.0004$) and over nephropathy by 24% (95% CI, 0.03-0.04; $P = 0.027$)	Ramipril reduces CVD events and nephropathy in high-risk diabetics
MIRACLE (Multicenter InSync Randomized Clinical Evaluation [North America])[1]	Randomized, exercise/QOL end point, clinical trial of atrial-biventricular pacing in NYHA-FC III/IV CHF patients with wide QRS but no indications for a pacemaker	Exercise performance and QOL improved with biventricular pacing	Mechanical approach to CHF may improve efficiency of cardiac contraction by resynchronization and decrease mitral regurgitation
MIRACLE ICD (Multicenter InSync Randomized Clinical Evaluation Implantable Cardioverter Defibrillator)[193,315]	Randomized, exercise/QOL end point, clinical trial of atrial-biventricular pacing with device having ICD capabilities in patients with indication for ICD but not a pacemaker	Similar findings as MIRACLE but in populations with ICD indications	Extends concepts of MIRACLE, but CHF patient applicability broadened by coupling ICD capabilities to cardiac resynchronization

5

Continued

Acronym (Full Title)	Study Design	Findings	Therapeutic Implication
MOCHA (Multicenter Oral Carvedilol Heart Failure Assessment)[39]	Placebo-controlled, dose-range study of carvedilol in mild-to-moderate stable HF (n = 345)	Dose-related improvements in LV function and dose-related reductions in mortality and hospitalization rates	Higher doses of carvedilol produce better outcomes
MOXCON (Moxonidine in Congestive Heart Failure)[40,285]	Mortality end point trial planned for ~4000 NYHA-FC II/IV CHF patients with EF <40%	Study terminated early because moxonidine associated with increase in mortality	Reasons for adverse outcomes not clear; concept of central α-blockade in HF may not deserve more scrutiny
MUSTIC (Multisite Stimulation in Cardiomyopathy)[55]	Randomized HF patients with no pacer indications to biventricular pacer on or off in crossover, single-blind design with 6″ walk primary end point (n = 58)	Biventricular pacer "on" group had greater increase in 6″ walk, peak VO₂, and QOL	Small, early clinical trial suggesting bi-ventricular pacing might be helpful in some CHF patients, but observations limited by design problems (crossover)
MUSTT (Multicenter Unsustained Tachycardia Trial)[44,201]	Randomized trial of EPS guided anti-arrhythmic therapy or simple HF treatment in CAD patients with EF <0.40 and asymptomatic NSVT; out-comes were SCD or cardiac arrest (n = 2202 with 1397 in a registry)	Mortality after 5 years was 48% with induc-ible VT vs 44% without (P = 0.005)	Study suggests that EPS identifies a high-risk group of CAD HF patients
Myocarditis Treatment Trial: A Clinical Trial of Immunosuppressive Therapy for Myocarditis[183]	Patients with biopsy-proven myocar-ditis and EF <0.45 randomly assigned (open-label) to standard care vs immunosuppression for 24 weeks with EF primary end point (n = 111)	No improvement noted with prednisone plus either cyclosporine or azathioprine therapy	Results did not support routine treat-ment of myocarditis with immuno-suppressive drugs

Study	Design	Findings	Comments
OPTIME-CHF (Outcomes of a Prospective Trial of Intravenous Milrinone for Exacerbations of Chronic Heart Failure)[105]	Multicenter, randomized, placebo-controlled trial of milrinone vs dobutamine in patients (n = 950) hospitalized for CHF management (decompensation not to point of requiring inotropes) to determine if LOS could be shortened	No impact on LOS outcomes; more adverse events with milrinone	Routinely prescribed inotropes may not be beneficial in CHF patients and could be associated with an increase in adverse events (new AF and sustained hypotension, $P < 0.05$); must distinguish between milrinone's use for very advanced CHF
OVERTURE (Omapatrilat vs Enalapril Randomized Trial of Utility in Reducing Events)[211]	5770 with NYHA II-IV CHF randomized to omapatrilat vs enalapril with death/CHF hospitalization primary end point	Omapatrilat not significantly better than enalapril in this population	ACEI/neutral endopeptidase combination not significantly better than ACEI alone in CHF
PIAF (Pharmacological Intervention in Atrial Fibrillation)[134]	Randomized trial of AF patients to diltiazem vs amiodarone (rate vs rhythm control) with symptomatic improvement primary end point; 17% had cardiomyopathy with symptoms primarily of palpitations, dyspnea (66%), and dizziness observed (n = 252)	23% of amiodarone group converted with 6" walk better but hospitalizations more frequent (69% vs 24%; $P = 0.001$) and more adverse drug events (25% vs 14%; $P = 0.036$)	Not much symptomatic difference between rate vs rhythm control, with exercise tolerance better, but more hospitalizations and problems with amiodarone (note few CHF patients)
PICO (Pimobendan in Congestive Heart Failure)[230]	Randomized, double-blind placebo-controlled trial of the PDE inhibitor pimobendan in CHF with exercise as primary end point (n = 317)	Pimobendan added to ACEI/diuretic improved exercise duration with no effect on VO_{2max} or QOL, with more deaths seen in the pimobendan group (RR, 1.8; 95% CI, 0.9-3.5)	Only slight improvement with this oral PDE inhibitor; potential for pro-arrhythmia concerning
PRAISE (Prospective Randomized Amlodipine Survival Evaluation)[104,217]	Effect of amlodipine, a long-acting calcium antagonist, vs placebo on survival against background of digoxin, diuretic, ACEI	Benefits seemed confined to dilated cardiomyopathy group; overall, drug seemingly well tolerated	Suggested at least one calcium channel blocker might be safe and possibly advantageous in select nonischemic CHF patients

5

Continued

Acronym (Full Title)	Study Design	Findings	Therapeutic Implication
PRAISE-II (Prospective Randomized Amlodipine Survival Evaluation-II)[104,217]	Randomized, multicenter, placebo-controlled, add-on amlodipine therapy in 1800 patients with dilated, nonischemic cardiomyopathy with mortality primary end point	No harm or benefit detected with amlodipine therapy	In a properly powered mortality end point clinical trial, the calcium channel blocker amlodipine did not confer benefit and negated suggestion of benefit in PRAISE-II
PRECISE/MOCHA (Prospective Randomized Evaluation of Carvedilol on Symptoms and Exercise/Multicenter Oral Carvedilol Heart Failure Assessment)[214]	Patients randomized to placebo vs carvedilol in three distinct subgroups to accommodate mild, moderate, or severe CHF; ascending carvedilol dose as tolerated (PRECISE) vs fixed dose carvedilol (MOCHA)	Trials combined with two others to suggest mortality reduction; effects on exercise tolerance minimal; clinical CHF improved (Carvedilol Program)	Carvedilol was first β-blocker (with α-blocking properties) to be given regulatory approbation for HF therapeutics
PRIME-II (Second Prospective Randomized Study of Ibopamine on Mortality and Efficacy)[121,178]	Placebo-controlled, mortality end point trial of a novel dopaminergic-1 active agent in 2200 advanced CHF patients	Trial stopped prematurely after 1906 patients because of excessive treatment-group mortality	Though drug has primary effects of peripheral and renal vasodilation without significant inotropic or pro-arrhythmia, there was a negative mortality impact; drug will not be developed in the United States
PROFILE (Prospective Randomized Flosequinan Longevity Evaluation)[195,242]	Effect of flosequinan vs placebo on survival against digoxin, diuretic, ACEI background	A higher mortality rate in the flosequinan group (100 mg/d) was observed compared with placebo	Forced withdrawal of flosequinan from the market in May 1993
PROMISE (Prospective Randomized Milrinone Survival Evaluation)[212,207]	Survival evaluation of milrinone vs placebo against digoxin, diuretic, ACEI background	Milrinone produced decreased survival and increased side effects compared with placebo	PDE inhibitors used chronically in HF likely to improve symptoms at the risk of higher mortality

PROVED (Prospective Randomized Study of Ventricular Failure and the Efficacy of Digoxin)[297,317]	Efficacy evaluation in patients with stable HF, on digoxin and diuretics, randomized to continued digoxin or withdrawal on placebo (same design as RADIANCE)	Digoxin-withdrawal group demonstrated significant deterioration of exercise tolerance and increased treatment failure	Small trial support for digoxin use in CHF (and caution against stopping drug)
RADIANCE (Randomized Assessment of Digoxin and Inhibitors of Angiotensin-Converting Enzyme)[215]	Patients with moderate-to-severe HF were randomized to remain on digoxin or be withdrawn on placebo	Patients withdrawn to placebo had deterioration of exercise performance and worsening symptoms compared with individuals maintained on digoxin	Triple therapy with ACEI, diuretic, and digoxin likely is best baseline approach to CHF treatment
RALES (Randomized Aldactone Evaluation Study)[29,236,251,304,322]	Randomized, multicenter, placebo-controlled mortality end point trial in 1663 NYHA-FC III/IV CHF patients over the age of 60 years	30% reduction in risk of death ($P < 0.001$) with low doses of aldactone	Older patients with more advanced CHF may benefit with aldactone added to other agents to more completely block the adverse neuro-hormonal milieu associated with HF; hyperkalemia could be a problem
REFLECT (Randomized Evaluation of Flosequinan on Exercise Tolerance)[216]	Randomized, double-blind exercise tolerance trial of the vasodilator flosequinan in NYHA-FC II/III patients	After 12 weeks, patients exercised better and symptomatically improved on flosequinan	Though flosequinan improved CHF symptoms, the excess mortality noted in the PROFILE study killed drug
REMATCH (Randomized Evaluation of Mechanical Assistance Therapy as an Alternative in Congestive Heart Failure)[254]	68 of 129 patients with end-stage HF and NYHA IV (most on IV inotropes) randomized to Heartmate LVAD vs optimal medical management	At 2 years, more LVAD patients alive (23% vs 8%; $P = 0.09$); morbidity cost (infection, bleeding, device malfunction) high	It is still unknown if this is a rational option for desperately ill CHF patients
RENAISSANCE (Randomized Etanercept North American Strategy to Study Antagonism of Cytokines)[89]	Randomized, composite end point, placebo-controlled, multicenter trial with twice weekly injections of TNF modulator added to standard therapies in NYHA-FC II/IV CHF patients with EF <30%	Trial stopped early because of apparent futility to answer hypothesis	Perhaps the wrong agent was chosen to test the "cytokine hypothesis"

5

Continued

113

Acronym (Full Title)	Study Design	Findings	Therapeutic Implication
RESOLVD (Randomized Evaluation of Strategies for Left Ventricular Dysfunction)[111,188,248,294]	Double-blind pilot study in which CHF patients randomized to candesartan (several doses), candesartan plus enalapril, or enalapril for a mean of 43 weeks with exercise tolerance, ventricular function, QOL, neurohormone levels, and tolerability of CHF end points ($n = 768$)	No differences noted in exercise, functional class, or QOL, but LV volumes better and BP and BNP levels lower with combination therapy	Candesartan as effective, safe, and tolerable as enalapril in CHF with candesartan/enalapril seemingly more beneficial for preventing remodeling than either drug alone
RESOLVD (Metoprolol Study) (Randomized Evaluation of Strategies for Left Ventricular Dysfunction–β-Blocker)[111,188,248,294]	During RESOLVD, long-acting metoprolol given in double-blind, factorial design fashion after initial up-titration of candesartan/enalapril with same RESOLVD end points ($n = 426$)	No differences in exercise, functional class, or QOL, but significant improvement of LV function and attenuation of remodeling with greater decrease of AII ($P = 0.036$) and renin levels ($P = 0.032$) but increase of BNP levels ($P < 0.01$) with long-acting metoprolol	When added to an ACE, ARB, or ACE/ARB combo, long-acting metoprolol improves LV function, reduces activation of renin-angiotensin system, and results in fewer deaths
RITZ (Randomized Intravenous Tezosentan)[291]	Prospective, randomized, double-blind, placebo-controlled, multicenter study of the ERA tezosentan in decompensated HF (hemodynamic end points) ($n = 285$)	Tezosentan proved a potent arteriolar vasodilator and reduced filling pressures as well with improving dyspnea	Parenteral ERA tezosentan may prove an effective agent in decompensated CHF
SAVE (Survival and Ventricular Enlargement)[227]	Effect of placebo vs captopril on survival and ventricular enlargement in LVD patients following MI	Captopril improved survival, functional status, and reduced repeat MI compared with placebo	Even in asymptomatic ventricular dysfunction postinfarct, ACEI beneficial
SCD-HeFT (Sudden Cardiac Death–Heart Failure Trial)[27]	CHF patients without AICD indications randomized to amiodarone, AICD, or routine CHF therapy with total mortality end point ($n = 2500$)	Trial ongoing	Study will likely clarify role of routine AICD or amiodarone therapy in CHF patients

SHOCK (Should We Emergently Revascularize Occluded Coronaries for Cardiogenic Shock)[131-133]	Randomized open study of early re-vascularization strategies (percutaneous and surgical) in patients with post-MI shock (86% on IABC) (n = 302)	Mortality at 30 days no different between medical and surgical groups, but 6-month mortality lower in latter (50% vs 63%; P = 0.027)	Early revascularization should be considered for MI patients with shock
SMILE (Survival of Myocardial Infarction: Long-Term Evaluation)[11]	Double-blind, placebo-controlled, multicenter, mortality end point evaluation of zofenopril postanterior MI (not eligible for thrombolytics) (n = 1556)	Risk reduction for death or severe CHF was 34% (95% CI, 0.08 - 0.54; P = 0.01) with routine zofenopril in this population	More evidence supporting routine ACEI use post-AMI
SOLVD (Studies of Left Ventricular Dysfunction) (treatment and prevention trials)[37,91,155,276-278,320]	Patients with symptomatic HF and decreased EF (treatment trial) or asymptomatic LVD (prevention trial) were randomized to placebo vs enalapril	Enalapril improved survival and symptoms in the treatment trial and delayed onset or progression of HF in the prevention trial	Taken together, trials established concept that ACEI is first-line therapy in all HF patients (not just CHF ones)
SPICE-Registry (Study of Patients Intolerant of Converting Enzyme Inhibitors [clinical registry])[28,109,259]	Multinational (8 countries) registry of patients (n = 9580) with CHF to determine medication utilization patterns and reasons for so-called ACEI intolerance	In optimal situations it seems that about 80% of CHF patients with depressed EF tolerate ACEI; in the 20% who do not, cough is the major reason for intolerance	In optimal circumstances, we should anticipate being able to get 80% of CHF patients with systolic LVD on ACEI
SPICE-Trial (Study of Patients Intolerant of Converting Enzyme Inhibitors [clinical trial])[28,109,259]	Double-blind, placebo-controlled, randomized clinical trial of candesartan to determine tolerability of an ARB in ACEI-intolerant patients (n = 270)	Over 12 weeks of study, statistically equivalent numbers of candesartan and placebo were continued (83% vs 87%)	ACEI-intolerant CHF patients seemingly tolerate the ARB candesartan over 80% of the time, with discontinuations being no more frequent than with placebo
STRETCH (Symptom, Tolerability, Response to Exercise Trial of Candesartan Cilexetil in Heart Failure)[252]	Multicenter, double-blind, parallel, group study of CHF patients on either candesartan or placebo for 12 weeks with changes in exercise, functional class, and dyspnea fatigue score index determined; ACEI, calcium channel blockers, β-blockers, and antiarrhythmics not permitted (n = 844)	In a CHF setting with mostly digoxin/diuretic/vasodilator background therapy, candesartan was well tolerated and improved HF symptoms	Candesartan appears effective in HF patients off of standard ACEI/β-blocker therapies

5

Continued

Acronym (Full Title)	Study Design	Findings	Therapeutic Implication
SUPPORT (Study to Understand Prognoses and Preferences for Outcomes and Risks of Treatment)[137]	Case-matching and propensity-score analysis done to evaluate RHC use in critically ill patients ($n = 5735$)	Observational study suggesting RHC associated with increased mortality in all but CHF patients	Difficult to extrapolate results to tailored hemodynamic management of CHF groups
SWORD (Survival With Oral d-Sotalol)[302]	Randomized, placebo-controlled, multi-center trial in patients with EF <40% and recent (6 to 42 days) or remote (>42 days) AMI ($n = 3121$)	Study stopped prematurely because of excess treatment mortality (5% vs 3% death rate; P <0.008) in sotalol group	Even an antiarrhythmic agent with only pure potassium channel-blocking effects has adverse outcome in HF patients
TRACE (Trandolapril Cardiac Evaluation)[151,289]	Double-blind, placebo-controlled, mortality end point clinical trial of trandolapril post-MI when EF was <0.35 ($n = 1749$)	Significant reduction in mortality noted on ACEI; RR reduction was 0.22 (95% CI, 0.67–0.91; $P = 0.001$)	Evidence supports use of ACEI post-MI when systolic LVD present
Val-HeFT (Valsartan Heart Failure Trial)[67,68]	Double-blind, placebo-controlled, multi-center trial of valsartan added on in ACEI patients (92%) with about 35% on β-blocker with all-cause mortality and combined mortality and morbidity end points ($n = 5010$)	Largest ARB trial reported to date with ARB/ACEI combination tested; no mortality benefit, seeming morbidity benefit, but this mostly limited to 7% not on ACEI; possible adverse interaction with patients on both ACEI and β-blockers	Question of ARB's role in CHF remains unanswered; valsartan may be beneficial for ACEI-intolerant patients
VALIANT (Valsartan in Acute Myocardial Infarction Trial)[298]	Double-blind, placebo-controlled comparison of valsartan, captopril, and their combinations after AMI ($n = 9249$)	Massive trial showing no difference between captopril and valsartan in post-MI CHF	ACEI remains first choice in post-MI CHF, but ARB valsartan is reasonable alternative

VEST (Vesnarinone Evaluation of Survival Trial)[65,95,96]	Large-scale, mortality end point trial of 60 mg and 30 mg doses in NYHA-FC III/IV patients on digoxin, diuretic, and ACEI	Increased mortality noted in contrast to prior study which suggested dramatic benefit	Role of vesnarinone in CHF in question; drug will not be pursued in the United States
V-HeFT-I (Vasodilator-Heart Failure Trial I)[64]	Parallel study of the effects of placebo, prazosin, and hydralazine on survival	Hydralazine/isosorbide dinitrate improved survival; prazosin was no different than placebo	First study to confirm that vasodilators could save lives in CHF
V-HeFT-II (Vasodilator-Heart Failure Trial II)[66]	Parallel study of enalapril vs hydralazine/isosorbide dinitrate on survival in moderate HF	Enalapril significantly improved survival; hydralazine/isosorbide dinitrate improved EF and exercise	First study to demonstrate incremental benefit of vasodilators with "endocrinologic" effect
V-HeFT-III (Vasodilator-Heart Failure Trial III)[5,35,69]	2 × 2 factorial-design study evaluating the efficacy of felodipine, digoxin, and placebo	No mortality reduction noted; felodipine seemingly well tolerated	Felodipine possibly another calcium channel-blocking drug that can be used safely in CHF, though not "beneficial"
VMAC (Vasodilation in the Management of Acute Congestive Heart Failure)[319]	Randomized, multicenter, nitroglycerin-controlled, symptom/hemodynamic end point clinical trial (n = 500) of nesiritide (BNP) infusion in severe CHF patients	BNP superior to nitroglycerin; better tolerated, and easier to use in decompensated CHF	Vasodilating efficacy of BNP in severe CHF demonstrated; VMAC designed to evaluate safety of different infusion strategies, including those not utilizing ICU/PAP monitoring
WATCH (Warfarin Anticoagulation Trial in CHF)[138,139]	Multicenter, randomized, placebo-controlled trial of anticoagulation vs platelet inhibition to reduce CHF morbidity/mortality	Trial ongoing	Study will clarify wisdom of routine anticoagulation strategies in CHF patients
Xamoterol: Xamoterol in Severe Heart Failure[309]	Survival end point evaluation in 516 CHF patients; placebo-controlled, multicenter, European	Xamoterol associated with higher mortality at 90-day point	Inotropic agents with β-agonist effects increase mortality in CHF patients

Continued

5

Abbreviations: AII, angiotension II; ACEI, angiotension-converting enzyme inhibitor; AF, atrial fibrillation; AICD, automatic implantable cardioverter defibrillator; AMI, acute myocardial infarction; ARB, angiotensin receptor blocker; ASCVD, arteriosclerotic cardiovascular disease; BNP, brain natriuretic peptide; BP, blood pressure; CABG, coronary artery bypass graft; CAD, coronary artery disease; CHF, congestive heart failure; CI, confidence interval; CV, cardiovascular; CVD, cardiovascular disease; EF, ejection fraction; EKG, electrocardiogram; EPS, electrophysiologic study; ERA, endothelin receptor antagonist; GH, growth hormone; GISSI-III, Gruppo Italiano per lo Studio della Sopravvivenza nell'Infarto miocardico-III; HF, heart failure; IABC, intraaortic balloon counterpulsation; ICD, implantable cardioverter defibrillator; ICU, intensive care unit; IDC, idiopathic dilated cadiomyopathy; ISIS-IV, Fourth International Study of Infarct Survival; IV, intravenous; IVIG, intravenous immunoglobulin; LOS, length of stay; LV, left ventricle; LVAD, left ventriclar assist device; LVD, left ventricular dysfunction; LVEF, left ventricular ejection fraction; MI, myocardial infarction; NSVT, nonsustained ventricular tachycardia; NYHA-FC, New York Heart Association functional class; PAP, pulmonary artery pressure; PDE, phosphodiesterase; PVC, premature ventricular contraction; QOL, quality of life; RHC, right-heart catheterization; RR, relative risk; SAEKG, signal-averaged electrocardiogram; SCD, sudden cardiac death; SMILE, Survival of Myocardial Infarction Long-Term Evaluation; TRACE, Trandolapril Cardiac Evaluation Study; VA, ventricular arrhythmia; VF, ventricular fibrillation; VO$_2$, volume of oxygen utilization; VO$_{2max}$, peak oxygen consumption; VT, ventricular tachycardia.

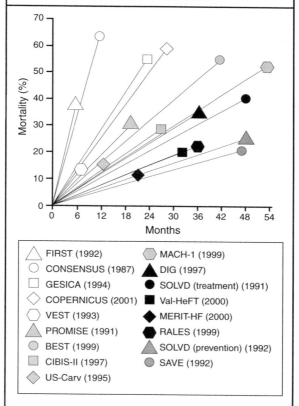

FIGURE 5.1 — CLINICAL HEART FAILURE TRIALS PLACEBO MORTALITY CURVES LINEARIZED

Legend:
- △ FIRST (1992)
- ○ CONSENSUS (1987)
- □ GESICA (1994)
- ◇ COPERNICUS (2001)
- ⬡ VEST (1993)
- ▲ PROMISE (1991)
- ● BEST (1999)
- ■ CIBIS-II (1997)
- ◆ US-Carv (1995)
- ⬡ MACH-1 (1999)
- ▲ DIG (1997)
- ● SOLVD (treatment) (1991)
- ■ Val-HeFT (2000)
- ◆ MERIT-HF (2000)
- ⬢ RALES (1999)
- ▲ SOLVD (prevention) (1992)
- ● SAVE (1992)

Abbreviations: BEST, β-Blocker Evaluation of Survival Trial; CIBIS-II, Cardiac Insufficiency Bisoprolol Study-II; CONSENSUS, Cooperative North Scandinavian Enalapril Survival Study; COPERNICUS, Carvedilol Prospective Randomized Cumulative Survival [trial]; DIG, Digitalis Investigation Group; FIRST, Flolan International Randomized Survival Trial; GESICA, Grupo de Estudio de la Sobrevida en la Insuficiencia Cardiaca en Argen-

Continued

tina; MACH-1, Mortality Assessment in Congestive Heart Failure I; MERIT-HF, Metoprolol CR/XL Randomized Intervention Trial in Heart Failure; PROMISE, Prospective Randomized Milrinone Survival Evaluation; RALES, Randomized Aldactone Evaluation Study; SAVE, Survival and Ventricular Enlargement; SOLVD, Studies of Left Ventricular Dysfunction; US-Carv, US Carvedilol Heart Failure Study; V-HeFT, Valsartan Heart Failure Trial; VEST, Vesnarinone Evaluation of Survival Trial.

The wide spectrum of mortality rates in placebo groups of select clinical trials performed over the past decade points to the heterogeneity of patient populations more than anything else. Once must always remember that when dealing with individual patients.

a massive undertaking that randomized almost 8000 HF patients into a study of digoxin against placebo.[84,106,209,284] Interestingly, this trial had a significant number of patients with diastolic dysfunction in the study (approximately 1,000 participants). CHARM, which was a trial involving an approximately 2500-patients with HF and EF >40%, was larger (the CHARM-Preserved Trial) and the only trial to date specifically designed and reported about this population. At the 5-year end point, digoxin did not have a significant impact on mortality but did reduce morbidity by diminishing HF hospitalizations. Observations were similar in patients having EFs >45%. Thus digoxin appears to be an important drug in patients with CHF and relatively preserved systolic LVD. This trial independently confirmed observations made in the smaller PROVED[297,317] and RADIANCE[215,317] studies, which were digoxin-withdrawal trials, focused on patients with clinically stable CHF. These three studies indicate that for symptomatic CHF, the baseline combination of diuretic, digoxin, and ACEIs is likely the best. These observations set the stage for gaining β-blocker add-on clinical trial experience.

β-Blocker Trials

Clinical trials of β-blockers in HF patients have now actually randomized more patients than the ACEI HF studies. The use of β-adrenergic blocking drugs has been controversial because of bradycardia and negative inotropy. Early on, the MDC Study compared the β_1-selective β-blocker metoprolol with placebo on top of background therapy with some end points suggesting benefit.[301] Subsequently, the carvedilol program, which initially was composed of four separate clinical trials pooled for morbidity and mortality results, demonstrated improvement in patients with mild-to-moderate compensated CHF when the β-blocker carvedilol was added to digoxin, diuretics, and ACEIs. Carvedilol is a nonselective β_1- and β_2-receptor antagonist and also is an α-adrenergic blocker. It is, therefore, a vasodilating β-blocker. More recent studies with other β-blockers have also demonstrated substantial morbidity and mortality reduction. CIBIS-I and II[61,62,101,160] using bisoprolol and MERIT-HF[129,191] using long-acting metoprolol were also positive β-blocker studies. In the United States, two β-adrenergic blocking drugs now have Food and Drug Administration (FDA) approval for use in HF patients: carvedilol (Coreg) and long-acting metoprolol (Toprol-XL).

COMET was a laudable effort to address the question of differential benefits in CHF patients between a β_1-selective receptor blocker (metoprolol) and a nonspecific β_1- and β_2-receptor blocker with α-blocking effects as well.[238] The trial was designed and initiated before MERIT-HF results with long-acting metoprolol were available and thus focused on the shorter-acting metoprolol at what some would now consider a low dose for HF patients, 50 mg twice daily (MERIT-HF had a target dose of 200 mg daily for the long-acting preparation). A total of 3029 patients (EF <35%) with chronic CHF (NYHA-FC II-IV) and a previous hospitalization for HF were randomized and followed for a mean of 58 months. With carvedilol, the mean heart rate reduction was 13 beats per minute and with metoprolol, 11.7 beats per minute, suggesting that β-blockade occurred in each group. All-cause mortality was 34% in the carvedilol-treated patients and 40% in the metoprolol group ($P = 0.0017$). The composite end point of all-cause mortality and all-cause hospital admission was not statistically significant in its difference (74% carvedilol vs 75% metoprolol; $P = 0.122$) nor was there a difference in the incidence of withdrawals for side effects.

COMET suggests that not all β-blockers or preparations are the same in CHF cohorts, particularly when taken in the context of BEST, which was neutral and showed no statistically significant morbidity/mortality reduction with bucindolol.[31] Only three β-blockers (carvedilol, metoprolol succinate, and bisoprolol) have shown consistent survival improvement, generally ranging around 35% of patients. COMET demonstrated that carvedilol 25 mg twice daily is superior to 50 mg metoprolol tartrate twice daily. It is not known if one agent or the other would prove to be better if the longer-acting metoprolol succinate preparation at the 200-mg daily dose was compared with carvedilol 25 mg twice daily.

Taken as a whole, the more recently completed studies of β-blockers support a treatment recommendation that counsels against using short-acting metoprolol tartrate and focuses on carvedilol or metoprolol succinate at the target doses of 25 mg twice daily or 200 mg once daily, respectively. Differences in bioavailability of metoprolol tartrate vs metoprolol succinate and dosing schedules used have fueled arguments about the details of some of the recently completed clinical trials involving β-blockers. Metoprolol succinate is 30% to 35% less bioavailable than metoprolol tartrate (meaning 150 mg of metoprolol succinate is equivalent to approximately 100 to 105 mg of metoprolol tartrate). It is unlikely that there will be a direct comparison of carvedilol vs metoprolol succinate to more definitely answer the question of superiority. In the meantime, clinicians have, at the very least, two effective β-blockers for use in CHF patients. Perhaps metoprolol succinate has the edge when treating patients with reactive airway disease or when a once-daily preparation is desired. Some would suggest that carvedilol should then be used in the remaining HF populations, including those with decreased EF and HF early post-MI (a contention supported by the most recent β-blocker postinfarction study, the CAPRICORN trial[50]).

Arrhythmia Trials

Malignant ventricular arrhythmias are frequent in patients with HF, but antiarrhythmic drugs have not fared well in clinical trials. CAST studied encainide, flecainide, and moricizine in post-MI patients with multiple premature ventricular contractions and systolic LVD.[51-53,119] Patients resembled those in the ACEI post-MI trials, but in contrast to those studies, CAST was terminated prematurely because of excessive mortality in all antiarrhythmic treatment groups. The SWORD trial evaluated the effect of *d*-sotalol mortality in patients with an EF >40% after MI and also had excessive treatment-group mortality.[302]

Amiodarone may be beneficial in HF. The GESICA trial was an unblinded, placebo-controlled, mortality end-point evaluation of amiodarone in moderate to severe HF and showed mortality and morbidity reduction.[86] The drug was stopped frequently, however, because of gastrointestinal and other side effects. EMIAT[142] and CAMIAT[47,48] are additional amiodarone HF trials suggesting that morbid arrhythmic events were reduced with routine amiodarone prescriptions. Both studies have been criticized, however, for drawing conclusions from end points that presumed ventricular arrhythmic death. An additional amiodarone study, the CHF-STAT, did not demonstrate a reduction in overall mortality. Although the data do not support prophylactic amiodarone therapy in HF patients to prevent mortality, these trials as a group did not suggest that amiodarone increased mortality. For HF patients requiring antiarrhythmic therapy for specific indications, amiodarone remains the most reasonable choice.

Two large studies of the newest antiarrhythmic drug, dofetilide, DIAMOND-CHF[150,290] and DIAMOND-MI[150,290] have recently been reported. Both trials had primary mortality end points. The CHF study assessed mortality in symptomatic CHF patients with severe LVD and the MI study randomized patients with severe LVD after MI. The CHF study did show that dofetilide decreased CHF hospitalization and converted atrial fibrillation but with a significant incidence of torsades de pointes in the antiarrhythmic group.

Because of the disappointment with the use of antiarrhythmic drugs, a number of studies have tried to clarify the role of implantable antiarrhythmic devices. MADIT evaluated the prophylactic use of an implanted cardioverter device (ICD) compared with conventional medical therapy in patients with prior infarction, a left ventricular EF <35%, and significant ventricular arrhythmia risk.[198] Mortality was significantly lower with the device than with conventional antiarrhythmic drugs. MADIT-II was a much larger mortality endpoint trial (discussed in more detail in Chapter 10, *Arrhythmia and Electrophysiologic Considerations*) that definitively demonstrated that routine ICD implantation saves lives in post-MI patients with dilated ventricles and low EF. This has led to radical changes in our approach to postinfarction patients with HF. Other defibrillator trials, some coupled with cardiac resynchronization therapies, designed to study both prophylactic implantations and therapeutic implantations (vs antiarrhythmic drugs), are ongoing. The more the data accumulate, the better these devices seem to be faring in this patient population. Nonetheless, precisely defining the patient population to benefit from device implantation is still a challenge.

Angiotensin Receptor Blocker Trials

Studies of angiotensin receptor blocking (ARB) agents are just now ending. These drugs generated great hope because they are so well tolerated. Some suggested that they could be an alternative to ACEIs; however, their mechanism of action is quite different from that of ACEIs. ELITE-I suggested that losartan was arguably a bit better tolerated than captopril in elderly HF patients who were beginning either an ACEI or an ARB.[153,231,234] Mortality was reduced in this trial, but this could not be confirmed in ELITE-II, a larger-scale and more properly designed mortality end-point trial of losartan.[93,153,232] The recently completed V-HeFT, which evaluated valsartan, likewise did not show a mortality reduction with this drug, but the combined morbidity/mortality end point was beneficially impacted.[67,68]

VALIANT, which was conducted in patients post-MI with HF, suggested equal morbidity and mortality benefits of valsartan compared with captopril.

The multiple CHARM trials have brought some closure to many vexatious questions regarding utility of ARBs, candesartan in particular, in patients with HF. CHARM was a program of four distinct trials with a fifth protocol-prespecified analysis of pooled data from the two trials entering patients with systolic LVD (EF <40%; CHARM-Alternative and CHARM-Added).[110,187,189,229,286,321]

The CHARM-Alternative trial randomized 2028 patients with symptomatic HF and low EF intolerant of ACEIs (mostly because of cough) to candesartan

125

(forced titration target dose 32 mg daily) or placebo. The unadjusted hazard ratio and 95% confidence interval (CI) for the primary end point of cardiovascular death or CHF hospitalization during a median follow-up of 33.7 months was 0.77, 0.67-0.89; P <0.0001. Each component of the end point was reduced as was the total number of hospital admissions for CHF.

The CHARM-Added trial randomized 2545 patients already on an ACEI (enalapril, mean equivalent dose about 17 mg daily which was close to the SOLVD Treatment Trial dose) to placebo or candesartan. Candesartan reduced the same primary end point by 15%; hazard ratio and 95% CI of 0.85, 0.75-0.95; $P = 0.011$.

In 3023 patients with EF >40%, candesartan was not associated with a reduction in cardiovascular mortality but did significantly reduce HF hospitalizations. In the combined analysis of patients in the CHARM-Added and CHARM-Alternative trials (patients with depressed EF), all primary and secondary end points were significantly reduced, including total mortality, cardiovascular mortality, and HF hospitalizations (as well as their combined end points). When all of the data were combined, there was a significant reduction in total mortality of 9%, $P = 0.032$ by analysis adjusted for prerandomization baseline differences. Importantly, these benefits were noted irrespective of the presence of a β-blocker or an aldosterone antagonist. These data clearly support the role of ARBs and, specifically, candesartan, in a broad spectrum of symptomatic HF patients irrespective of baseline EF or concomitant treatment with ACEIs, β-blockers, or aldosterone antagonists.

Trials of Other Approaches

Studies with calcium channel blockers generally have demonstrated increased morbidity and mortality in HF. PRAISE-I and II[104,217] and V-HeFT-III[15,35,69] are the only clinical trials to date that suggest that specific calcium channel blocking agents (amlodipine and felodipine) might not carry such concerns for CHF patients. The calcium channel blocker mibefradil studied in MACH-I increased morbidity. This drug is not available.

Several clinical trials with mortality end points have shown that some agents actually improve hemodynamics and symptoms in HF but increase morbidity. Examples of such studies are PROFILE (flosequinan),[195,242] PICO (pimobendan),[230] PROMISE (oral milrinone),[207,212] PRIME-II (ibopamine),[121,178] VEST (vesnarinone),[65,95,96] and Xamoterol (xamoterol).[309] Chronic oral therapy with milrinone, a phosphodiesterase inhibitor with inotropic and vasodilating properties, improved hemodynamics and clinical findings in HF patients, yet significantly increased mortality (generally, sudden cardiac death). Chronic orally administered flosequinan, another inotropic vasodilator (with primarily vasodilating properties), provided symptomatic improvement but increased mortality rates. The same can be said for vesnarinone, a drug that was studied with great hope after preliminary trials suggested that the agent was beneficial.

Other approaches in HF have been studied or are being evaluated in large-scale ongoing trials. Human growth hormone seemingly has some beneficial effects, but concern has been raised about the induction of ventricular hypertrophy and diastolic dysfunction with this agent. Spironolactone proved quite efficacious in the RALES trial when added to a regimen of diuretics, digoxin, and ACEIs in NYHA-FC II/III patients.[29,236,251,304,322] EPHESUS expanded on this observation with eplerenone, a new aldosterone antagonist that does not cause painful gynecomastia.[233,235] In an early post-MI population with LVD and HF, adding eplerenone to ACEIs and β-blockers decreased mortality.

Other treatment strategies under evaluation include surgery for coronary heart disease, aerobic exercise training, anticoagulation, and early right heart catheterization in critically ill patients. As these clinical trials are completed, even more information will be available to clinicians.

Summary

Table 5.2 and **Table 5.3** summarize what we have learned from over 2 decades of clinical trials focused on HF therapeutics. We now know that direct-acting vasodilating drugs relieve symptoms, but do not dramatically decrease mortality. Many trials have confirmed ACEIs as the primary option to improve outcomes in patients with either asymptomatic systolic LVD or frank CHF. ACEIs also benefit patients after acute MI, particularly those with systolic LVD or symptomatic CHF. ARBs have proven an attractive option for HF patients who cannot tolerate ACEIs, and their combination with ACEIs and β-blockers has proven valuable. These drugs may, at least, be equivalent to ACEIs.

Carvedilol, a β-adrenergic blocking agent (non-selective) with vasodilating properties, benefits patients with mild-to-moderate CHF when added to ACEI, digoxin, and diuretic therapy. Recently, the COPERNICUS trial confirmed that even in more seriously ill HF patients (stable, noncongested, NYHA-FC IV individuals), the drug is beneficial.[213] The CAPRICORN trial suggests that carvedilol is also helpful post-MI when HF is present.[50] Long-acting metoprolol, a β_1-selective β-blocker, has also proven effective in mild-to-moderate CHF patients, as has bisoprolol. Other β-blockers have not been well studied in HF or have not demonstrated the same benefits (eg, bucindolol in BEST[31]).

Amiodarone may be the most reasonable option when antiarrhythmic drugs are necessary in HF patients. Automatic cardioverter defibrillating devices will likely be the preferred tactic for HF complicated by potentially malignant ventricular arrhythmias. Digoxin remains an important drug for reduction of morbidity in HF patients; other positive inotropic agents for chronic oral therapy such as pimobendan, ibopamine, milrinone, and vesnarinone may actually increase sudden cardiac death syndrome rates. Although some studies have suggested detrimental effects of calcium channel blocking drugs in HF, amlodipine and felodipine may be exceptions. These drugs are not associated with increased mortality and morbidity but do not reduce these important end points. When other agents that are beneficial in HF, such as ACEIs and β-blockers, have failed to control hypertension or angina pectoris, amlodipine or felodipine may be safe adjuvants.

5

Clinical trials have given us great insight with regard to benefit or harm with certain therapeutic strategies. Ongoing trials will shape future treatment algorithms for HF patients. The vast majority of clinical trials have focused on the stable outpatient with CHF and few data are currently available regarding inpatient management of decompensated patients. This, we hope, will soon be corrected.

6 General Treatment Approaches

Heart failure (HF) therapy has become more complex but effective over the past 25 years. Accurate diagnosis and careful clinical staging of the HF patient provide the basis for determining treatment strategy. The initial management for each patient will be based on either prevention or treatment protocols, and subsequent management will follow as dictated by serial reassessments. The new American College of Cardiology/American Heart Association (ACC/AHA) HF stages expand the concept of the older New York Heart Association (NYHA) classification to include patients at risk for HF and emphasize prevention (**Figure 6.1**). As patients develop symptomatic HF, the NYHA classification helps to focus attention on candidates for increasingly intensive management, interventions, and devices. In asymptomatic or mildly symptomatic (New York Heart Association functional class [NYHA-FC] I/II) patients, we attempt to prevent progression of ventricular remodeling and forestall the appearance of symptoms. In more symptomatic patients (NYHA-FC III/IV), treatment should focus on:

- Reducing/eliminating the patient's symptoms
- Preventing further deterioration of ventricular function
- Reducing mortality.

Staging the severity of the HF syndrome by assigning or assessing ACC/AHA stage and NYHA-FC at each patient encounter is critical to this approach. As part of that process, one must determine if asymptomatic systolic left ventricular dysfunction (LVD) is

FIGURE 6.1 — PHILOSOPHY OF HEART FAILURE THERAPY

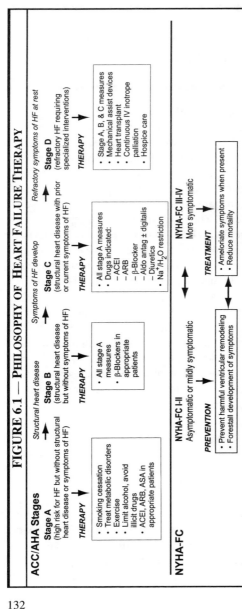

ACC/AHA Stages

Structural heart disease → *Symptoms of HF develop* → *Refractory symptoms of HF at rest*

Stage A
(high risk for HF but without structural heart disease or symptoms of HF)

THERAPY
- Smoking cessation
- Treat metabolic disorders
- Exercise
- Limit alcohol, avoid illicit drugs
- ACEI, ARB, ASA in appropriate patients

Stage B
(structural heart disease but without symptoms of HF)

THERAPY
- All stage A measures
- β-Blockers in appropriate patients

Stage C
(structural heart disease with prior or current symptoms of HF)

THERAPY
- All stage A measures
- Drugs indicated:
  – ACEI
  – ARB
  – β-Blocker
  – Aldo antag ± digitalis
  – Diuretics
  – Na⁺/H₂O restriction

Stage D
(refractory HF requiring specialized interventions)

THERAPY
- Stage A, B, & C measures
- Mechanical assist devices
- Heart transplant
- Continuous IV inotrope palliation
- Hospice care

NYHA-FC

NYHA-FC I-II
Asymptomatic or mildly symptomatic

PREVENTION
- Prevent harmful ventricular remodeling
- Forestall development of symptoms

NYHA-FC III-IV
More symptomatic

TREATMENT
- Ameliorate symptoms when present
- Reduce mortality

Abbreviations: ACC/AHA, American College of Cardiology/American Heart Association; ACEI, ACE inhibitor; aldo antag, aldosterone antagonist; ARB, angiotensin receptor blocker; ASA, acetylsalicylic acid; HF, heart failure; H₂O, water; IV, intravenous; Na⁺, sodium; NYHA-FC, New York Heart Association Functional Class.

Patients should receive therapeutics for heart failure based on either a prevention or treatment philosophy. In asymptomatic patients, strategies should be used to prevent development of ventricular remodeling progression and forestall the rise of symptoms. In symptomatic patients, treatment should focus on ameliorating the symptoms, preventing deterioration, and reducing mortality.

Modified from: Hunt SA, et al. *J Am Coll Card.* 2001;38:2101-2113.

6

present. This is important because a diagnosis of HF does not always mean congestion is present. Today's therapeutic approach to HF varies with severity (**Figure 6.1** and **Table 6.1**). Key to treating many patients with HF is recognizing the underlying disease processes that have caused the condition or precipitated symptoms. It is worth reemphasizing that HF is actually a syndrome or milieu and not a specific disease process. By identifying underlying primary diseases and comorbidities, one sets the stage for eliminating them if at all possible. Linked to this is determination of exacerbating factors, such as concurrent infections, medication noncompliance, or dietary indiscretion. With identification of important primary and exacerbating disease is consideration of surgical options, when appropriate.

Agents With Potential Adverse Effects in Heart Failure

Heart failure drug programs tend to involve multiple medications, and HF patients often have significant comorbidities. Most patients with HF present are already following a prescription (or nonprescription) drug program. A careful, evidence-based critical review of the previously prescribed drugs constitutes the first step in effective HF management. Drugs that have no proven benefit or are actually detrimental must be discontinued, with a reasonable explanation to the patient (and the prescribing physician). For example, most antiarrhythmic agents in HF have untoward proarrhythmic or other harmful effects. The same applies to most calcium channel blockers (felodipine and amlodipine are probably acceptable). Certain oral hypoglycemic agents, such as the insulin-sensitizing compounds rosiglitazone (Avandia) and pioglitazone (Actose), have the potential for increasing weight gain and fluid retention. Proper use of these drugs is yet to be clari-

134

TABLE 6.1 — HEART FAILURE THERAPEUTICS: GENERAL PRINCIPLES

- Make or confirm appropriate diagnosis:
  - Dyspnea, edema, and rales are not always indicative of congestive heart failure (CHF)
- Stage syndrome severity; assign or assess NYHA-FC at each visit (see **Table 4.10**):
  - Discover asymptomatic left ventricular systolic dysfunction
  - Note that heart failure (HF) does not always mean CHF
  - Note that therapeutic approaches to HF varies with severity of syndrome
- Treat underlying diseases:
  - Address etiologic problems if at all possible
  - Eliminate exacerbating factors
  - Consider surgical options when appropriate
- Stop drugs that have no proven benefit or that are potentially detrimental:
  - Most antiarrhythmic agents
  - Most calcium channel blockers
  - Certain oral hypoglycemic agents (thiazolidinedione compounds rosiglitazone/pioglitazone)
  - Nonsteroidal anti-inflammatory agents
  - Tricyclic antidepressants
  - Antihistaminics
  - Many dietary supplements such as ephedra and ephedra-containing compounds
- Begin therapeutic regimens with proven efficacy (titrate drug doses to targets):
  - Drugs to prevent functional deterioration:
    › ACE inhibitors
    › β-Blockers
  - Drugs to reduce mortality:
    › ACE inhibitors
    › ARBs
    › β-Blockers
    › Aldosterone antagonists
    › Hydralazine/isosorbide dinitrate

6

Continued

- Drugs to control symptoms:
  › Diuretics
  › Digoxin
  › ACE inhibitors
  › ARBs
  › β-Blockers
• Prescribe rational polypharmacy:
  - Use only drugs of proven benefit
  - Stop unnecessary agents
  - Stop potentially harmful agents
  - Use drugs with fewest side effects possible
  - Design program to ensure compliance (use once-daily drugs if possible)
  - Consider timing of drug administration (ie, give once-daily ACE inhibitor in AM and once daily β-blocker in PM if appropriate)
  - Consider cost of drugs employed
• Remember nonpharmacologic approaches:
  - Low-salt diet
  - Fluid restriction
  - Avoid nicotine and alcohol
  - Cardiac rehabilitation and aerobic exercise training

Abbreviations: ACE, angiotensin-converting enzyme; NYHA-FC, New York Heart Association functional class.

fied in patients with ventricular dysfunction; however, they are attractive agents because of beneficial endothelial effects. Further evaluations will help to clarify their risk:benefit ratios. Likewise, nonsteroidal anti-inflammatory drugs (NSAIDs) contribute to fluid retention and renal dysfunction in patients with HF. Tricyclic antidepressants and antihistaminics can also adversely affect the myocardium directly or increase afterload. β-Adrenergic blocking agents play extraordinarily important roles in HF patients, but some unstable and severely congested patients are worsened when exposed to these compounds. The use of anticoagulants solely because a patient has a low ejection fraction (EF) is controversial. Warfarin therapy to prevent vascular and embolic events in HF is currently under evaluation. Finally, it is coming to light that some dietary supplements are harmful, particularly those containing ephedra and its congeners; they must be avoided.

Evidence-Based Drug Therapy

Fortunately, physicians who manage patients with HF now have extensive data from clinical trials to support recommendations for pharmacologic management. The potent neurohormonal blocking agents, including angiotensin-converting enzyme inhibitors (ACEIs) and angiotensin receptor blockers (ARBs), β-blockers, and aldosterone antagonists, have all been shown to prevent functional deterioration, improve symptoms, and reduce intermediate-term mortality. β-Blockers have proven effects even in patients with advanced HF. Vasodilating regimens with hydralazine and isosorbide dinitrate can provide significant hemodynamic benefit in those who are truly ACEI intolerant, and may be combined with β-blockers and antialdosterone agents for some degree of neurohormonal blockade. Better yet, it has recently been demonstrated that some ARBs (valsartan and candesartan) fare as well as ACEI with respect to morbidity and mortality reduction in ACEI-intolerant patients. The results of the CHARM-Alternative Trial and V-HeFT confirmed this and although V-HeFT suggested a potential detrimental interaction when valsartan, an ACEI, and a β-blocker were combined, this was not the case in CHARM where candesartan was the ARB employed.[73,110,189,229,286,321] Both spironolactone and eplerenone have also demonstrated mortality reduction in elderly NYHA-FC III and IV congestive heart failure (CHF) patients (spironolactone in patients with HF more generally and eplerenone in those post–myocardial infarction [MI]).[29,235,322] Drugs to control symptoms of CHF include diuretics and digoxin, particularly

137

when added to ACEIs, ARBs, β-blockers, and a combination of hydralazine and isosorbide dinitrate.

Because treatment protocols are complicated, prescribing rational polypharmacy becomes important. We again emphasize using only drugs of proven benefit and stopping unnecessary or potentially harmful agents. Using drugs with the fewest side effects in any given individual is likewise important. Designing programs that ensure compliance (that is, using once- or twice-daily drugs if possible) is preferable. We favor administering both β-blockers and ACEIs twice daily between 6 AM and 7 AM and again 12 hours later. Using long-acting drugs on a twice-daily schedule helps to maintain around-the-clock neurohormonal suppression without escape. Orthostatic symptoms should be addressed by first carefully evaluating the importance of the symptoms. Is the lightheadedness causing functional impairment or is it just a nuisance? Often, support hosiery and flexing the calf muscles immediately on standing will suffice to relieve the symptoms. A reminder to the patient about the survival benefits of appropriate drug programs also puts many issues in perspective. If orthostatic issues are truly bothersome, the first therapeutic strategy is always reduction of diuretic doses if congestion is under control. Although diuretics are useful in HF management, both the patient and physician should clearly understand their risks and benefits. Diuretics do not improve outcome in HF; in fact, diuretic therapy tends to activate the renin-angiotensin system and might even exacerbate the pathophysiology of advanced HF. In the SOLVD database, patients with comparable disease severity fared better when managed without diuretics as compared with those who used daily doses. Modest doses of diuretics, preferably used intermittently in response to an increase in morning body weight, allow a more tolerable diet and improve quality of life. However, the life-saving therapeutic agents, either β-blockers or ACEI/

ARB agents, should not be discontinued or withheld because of diuretic-induced hypotension.

Though controversial, some evidence from long-term observations favors the use of warfarin in patients with LVD)[9] A recent cohort analysis from the SOLVD database showed improved survival and reduced morbidity in warfarin-treated patients due primarily to reduction in cardiac events. Further delineation of the population at risk will be important to optimizing the risk-benefit decisions involved. The likelihood of an oral thrombin inhibitor becoming available in the near future also promises that chronic oral anticoagulation in HF patients will remain a topic of active clinical study.

Nonpharmacologic Therapies

In addition to considering surgical interventions for primary diseases causing HF, one should not forget the importance of nonpharmacologic approaches to these patients. At the root of these strategies are:

- Low-sodium diet
- Fluid restriction in patients who are at risk for congestion
- Absolute smoking cessation
- Avoidance of alcohol
- Cardiac rehabilitation and regular exercise protocols.

Interestingly, many clinicians today still actively discourage exercise in patients with HF. This probably reflects the lingering influence of Dr. George Burch who advocated prolonged bedrest for patients with dilated cardiomyopathy.[41] As late as 1968, the noted British clinician, Dr Paul Wood (memorialized in the Wood unit for pulmonary resistance) also stated "rest in bed or in a comfortable armchair is essential and should be continued for a minimum period of 3 weeks," in the treatment of HF. The improved outcomes with modern drug therapy suggest that drugs today may be accomplishing what bedrest did yesterday, ie, reduction of neurohormonal activation.[191] Randomized trials have clearly demonstrated the benefit of aerobic exercise in well-managed HF patients.

Nonpharmacologic approaches to HF therapy are summarized in **Table 6.2**. They include the need for salt and water restriction, which may require extensive dietary counseling, and the need for caloric restriction, with weight loss to an appropriate body mass index. These issues, which are often critical to success in HF management, are frequently not addressed. In our experience, it is not unusual to have patients referred for cardiac transplantation before the first referral to a dietitian! Again, a candid discussion with patients regarding dietary modification is critical. In essence, the HF patient must understand that salt and water not ingested do not have to be removed with diuretics. Many HF patients can participate in significant levels of activity as alluded to previously. A functional assessment and appropriate rehabilitation strategy must be prescribed in order to maintain peripheral vascular tone, muscle mass, and good emotional health.

Counseling

When the diagnosis of HF is established, the physician (or other members of the HF team) must review educational issues with the patient and his or her family or other significant support. Suggested topics for counseling are listed in **Table 6.3**. Of course, patients will want to know what HF is and the reason for symptoms. The term "heart failure" is troubling because of its terribly negative connotation. After all, no one likes to fail at anything. Nonetheless, no better term is available. The probable cause of HF should be discussed,

TABLE 6.2 — NONPHARMACOLOGIC APPROACHES TO HEART FAILURE THERAPY

- Low-salt diets:
  - 3-g sodium diet for mild HF (NYHA-FC I/II)
  - 2-g sodium diet for more advanced HF (NYHA-FC III/IV)
- Fluid restriction:
  - <2000 cc/d when congestion present
  - <1500 cc/d when serum sodium <135 mEq/mL
- Daily weight:
  - Early morning weight:
    › Record daily or every other day
    › Use same scale on solid surface
    › Wear no clothing when weighing
- Prescribe cardiac rehabilitation:
  - Phase II program if not homebound
  - Home health consult if homebound
- Patient education:
  - Diet
  - Fluid restriction
  - Activity
  - Medications
  - Signs and symptoms of deterioration

Abbreviation: HF, heart failure; NYHA-FC, New York Heart Association functional class.

and expected symptoms, particularly symptoms of worsening HF, must be clarified. This discussion should be coupled with education about strategies to take if symptoms worsen. Patients must learn self-monitoring techniques: daily weighing, blood pressure, pulse rate, and blood glucose in diabetics. A specific explanation of the treatment and care plan is warranted. This is particularly important since some treatments may actually cause worsening of symptoms early on, yet effect substantive improvement weeks or months down the road. Furthermore, in asymptomatic patients, one must carefully explain the rationale for taking

TABLE 6.3 — EDUCATION AND COUNSELING: SUGGESTED TOPICS FOR PATIENT, FAMILY, AND CAREGIVER

- Explanation of heart failure (HF) and the reason for symptoms
- Cause or probable cause of HF
- Expected symptoms
- Symptoms of worsening HF
- What to do if symptoms worsen
- Self-monitoring with:
  - Daily weighing
  - Blood pressure
  - Pulse rate
  - Blood glucose (in diabetics)
- Explanation of treatment/care plan
- Clarification of patient's responsibilities
- Importance of cessation of tobacco and limitation of alcohol use
- Importance of dietary restrictions
- Role of family members or other caregivers in the treatment/care plan (eg, cardiopulmonary resuscitation [CPR] training)
- Availability and value of qualified local support group
- Importance of obtaining vaccinations against influenza and pneumococcal disease
- Sexual activity/use of sildenafil (Viagra)

medications when symptoms are absent. Clarification of a patient's responsibilities is also important, particularly as it relates to:

- Cessation of tobacco use
- Limitation of alcohol consumption (if appropriate)
- Low-sodium diet and fluid restriction plans.

The role of family members or other caregivers in the treatment process should also be delineated. Consider recommending formal cardiopulmonary resuscitation education. In many locales, qualified local support groups are available and sometimes of value. We stress the importance of obtaining vaccinations against influenza and pneumococcal disease. Both men and women appreciate a frank discussion of sexual activity and use of drugs that may be problematic, such as sildenafil (Viagra) and its newer iterations.

During the patient education process, a realistic discussion of the prognosis for individuals with HF must be undertaken, difficult as this may be. Patients need this information to place interventions into an appropriate context of risk and benefit. **Figure 6**.2 shows data from the Framingham Study for death rates for HF in various age groups related to gender and race. In addition, certain findings predict higher risk of early death (**Figure 6**.3). Lower EF and cardiac index with higher cardiac filling pressures are associated with worse outcomes. Objective measurement of metabolic exercise capabilities utilizing tools to quantify maximal O_2 consumption is extremely important. Patients with peak oxygen consumption (VO_{2max}) of <10 mL O_2 kg/min portends a poor prognosis (**Figure 4**.3). Documented ventricular tachycardia or atrial fibrillation (AF) worsens prognosis, as do high resting heart rate and low serum sodium.

Special Considerations in Heart Failure Due to Coronary Disease

Ischemic heart disease due to atherosclerotic obstruction of the major epicardial vessels occurs in approximately 40% of adults with HF. Extensive clinical data now support an aggressive approach to the diagnosis and treatment of myocardial ischemia in such patients. Multiple clinical trials have demonstrated that individuals with HF and viable but ischemic myocardium fare substantially better with direct revascularization. **Figure 6**.4 is one approach to evaluation and treatment of coronary artery disease in patients with HF. This schema was recommended as part of the first

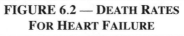

FIGURE 6.2 — DEATH RATES FOR HEART FAILURE

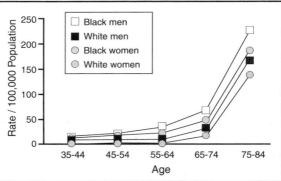

Death rates from heart failure increase substantially as the population ages.

McKee PA, et al. *N Engl J Med*. 1971;285:1441-1446.

formal position paper and treatment guidelines published for HF patient management. These Agency for Health Care Policy and Research (AHCPR) guidelines first ask the clinician to consider whether contraindications to revascularization might or might not be present. If not, one should counsel the patient to consider formal evaluation for ischemic heart disease and active ischemia to determine if revascularization is possible. In the patient with angina pectoris, one should proceed to coronary angiography in the hope that targets for revascularization are present. One must remember that overt chest pain might not always be present. Anginal equivalents are sometimes present as symptoms of CHF, particularly flash pulmonary edema and sudden inexplicable dyspnea. In the individual with no angina but a previous MI, evaluation for potentially viable myocardium that can benefit from revascularization strategies is mandatory. In individuals with no angina, no prior MI, but risk factors for

FIGURE 6.3 — RISK OF DEATH IN HEART FAILURE PATIENTS

	Lower Risk	Higher Risk
Ejection fraction	>0.4	<0.2
Cardiac index (L/min/m^2)	>2.5	<2.0
PCWP (mm Hg)	<16	>20
VO_{2max} (mL/kg/min)	>20	<10
Heart rhythm	Sinus	Documented ventricular or atrial fibrillation (either paroxysmal or sustained)
Heart rate	<80	>100
Serum Na+ (mmol/L)	>135	<135

Abbreviations: PCWP, pulmonary capillary wedge pressure; VO_{2max}, peak oxygen consumption.

Broadly summarized, as the ejection fraction and cardiac index fall, PCWP increases and volume of oxygen utilization (VO_2) maximum declines, the risk of death becomes higher. Arrhythmias and serum sodium simply magnify the likelihood of adverse outcome when present.

atherosclerotic cardiovascular disease, noninvasive ischemic heart disease evaluation should be considered.

Determining myocardial viability in individuals with chronic ischemic disease has become extraordinarily important. Many patients have akinetic ventricular segments that will revert to reasonable function with revascularization. The assessment of myocardial viability can involve any one of a number of approaches, including a combination of perfusion and metabolic imaging, assessment with dobutamine stress echocardiography, or evaluation with magnetic resonance imaging (MRI). These strategies are summarized in **Table 6.4**. Clinicians must choose the evaluation strat-

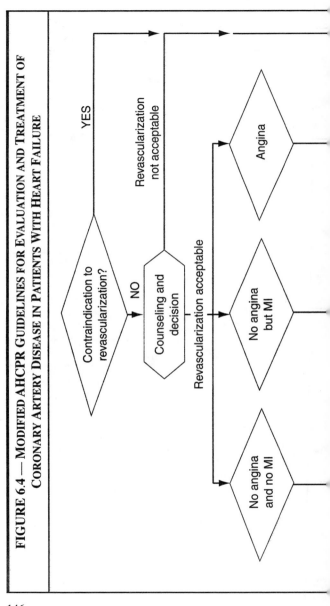

FIGURE 6.4 — MODIFIED AHCPR GUIDELINES FOR EVALUATION AND TREATMENT OF CORONARY ARTERY DISEASE IN PATIENTS WITH HEART FAILURE

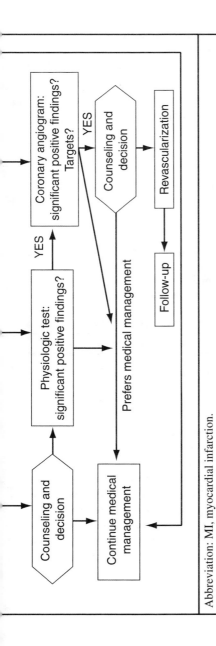

Abbreviation: MI, myocardial infarction.

The Agency for Health Care Policy and Research (AHCPR) guildeines focus on coronary artery disease in patients with heart failure because of the demonstrated benefit that revascularization may effect in some congestive heart failure patients with coronary artery disease.

147

TABLE 6.4 — APPROACHES TO IDENTIFYING VIABILITY IN HIBERNATING MYOCARDIUM

- Assessment of regional myocardial function using radionuclide methods, echocardiography, or magnetic resonance imaging during or after:
  - Nitroglycerin
  - Post extrasystolic potentiation
  - Catecholamine infusion (dobutamine)
  - Exercise
- Assessment of perfusion, membrane integrity, and metabolism:
  - TI-201 scintigraphy:
    › Rest-early redistribution-late redistribution
    › Exercise—redistribution/reinjection
  - Technetium 99m sestamibi
  - Positron emission tomography:
    › Flow: rubidium-82
    › Metabolism: fluorine-18 fluorodeoxyglucose, carbon-11 acetate
  - Magnetic resonance spectroscopy with gadolinium

Modified from: Castro PF, et al. *Am J Med.* 1998;104:69-79.

egy most likely to be productive with the technology available.

Anatomic information delineating the extent and severity of coronary pathology can be easily and safely obtained from diagnostic coronary arteriography. In our practice, we often omit left ventriculography at the time of coronary angiographic study to reduce the contrast burden and thus reduce the risk of contrast-induced nephropathy. With such an approach, adequate evaluation of coronary anatomy rarely requires large contrast doses or causes substantial renal dysfunction, even in patients with relatively advanced HF. If the coronary anatomy is suitable for percutaneous or direct surgical revascularization, a viability assessment is indicated using whatever techniques are available. The receiver-operating characteristic curves for sensitivity and specificity of most assessment technologies are remarkably similar. The challenge then becomes to determine which patient will benefit from revascularization. Clearly, those with active ischemia should be revascularized. In individuals with asymptomatic hibernating myocardium and extremely poor LV systolic function, our practice favors revascularization when the estimated total of ischemic plus hibernating myocardium approaches 20% of the left ventricle and, certainly, when higher.

Electrophysiologic Management

6

Chapter 10, *Arrhythmia and Electrophysiologic Considerations*, treats the electrophysiology of HF in detail, with emphasis on evidence-based management of electrical instability. Arrhythmia management and other facets of HF management should proceed in a coordinated fashion, with overall strategy and direction supervised by the cardiologist directing HF care. A close relationship with an electrophysiologist is essential because arrhythmias in HF are frequent and potentially disastrous. HF is an arrhythmogenic state with structural heart disease providing the substrate and neurohormonal activation the stimulus for serious electrical instability. **Table 6.5** emphasizes this fact by demonstrating the high incidence of sudden cardiac death (SCD) in several clinical trials. SCD often reflects an unstable ventricular arrhythmia that might be treated with medications or therapeutic defibrillating devices. **Table 6.6** indicates that the mechanism of sudden death in HF can be wide ranging, with all deaths necessarily being preventable by known therapeutic modalities. Ventricular tachycardia and fibrillation, however, are often noted in acute coronary syndromes, in the presence of ventricular scar where reentry arrhythmias can occur, or as torsades de pointes due

TABLE 6.5 — INCIDENCE OF SUDDEN DEATH IN HEART FAILURE CLINICAL TRIALS					
Study	Year Published	N	Mean Follow-up (mo)	Total Mortality (%)	SCD Mortality (%)
V-HeFT-I	1986	642	41	44	44
CONSENSUS	1987	253	6	38	25
V-HeFT-II	1991	804	30	35	36
SOLVD (treatment)	1991	2569	24	38	23
SOLVD (prevention)	1992	4228	37	15	31

Abbreviations: CONSENSUS, Cooperative North Scandanavian Enalapril Survival Study; SOLVD, Studies of Left Ventricular Dysfunction; SCD, sudden cardiac death; V-HeFT, Vasodilator-Heart Failure Trial.

TABLE 6.6 — MECHANISM OF SUDDEN DEATH IN HEART FAILURE

Event	Rhythm
Acute coronary syndrome	VT/VF
Ventricular scar reentry	VT
Torsades de pointes	VT
Sinus node/conduction system disease	Bradycardia/complete heart block
Metabolic derangement	VT, bradycardia, EMD
Pulmonary embolus	EMD
Cerebral vascular accident	Bradycardia
Aortic aneurysm rupture	EMD

Abbreviations: EMD, electromechanical dissociation; VF, ventricular fibrillation; VT, ventricular tachycardia.

to acute ischemia or adverse drug reactions. Metabolic derangements can account for ventricular tachycardia, bradycardia, and electromechanical dissociation. Sinus node dysfunction can cause bradycardia and heart block that results in SCD syndrome. Sudden death can also occur in the setting of an acute pulmonary embolus, cerebral vascular accident, or aortic aneurysm rupture, and these situations will not be influenced by an automatic internal cardioverting-defibrillating device or antiarrhythmic drugs.

Figure 6.5 emphasizes that the causes of arrhythmias in HF are multifactorial. HF provides an anatomic substrate favorable to arrhythmia, with left atrial and LV dilation, anatomic scarring, and stretching of the myocardial tissue. A neurohumoral environment favorable to arrhythmia with high sympathetic tone and renin-angiotensin system activation can be present. The pharmacologic environment can also favor arrhythmias

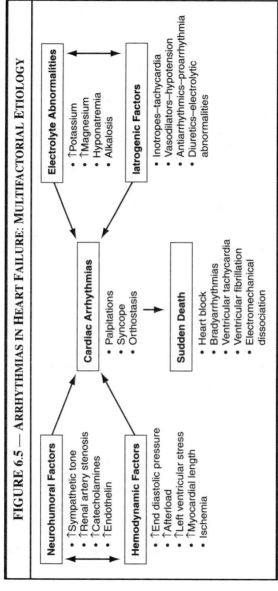

FIGURE 6.5 — ARRHYTHMIAS IN HEART FAILURE: MULTIFACTORIAL ETIOLOGY

Neurohumoral Factors
• ↑Sympathetic tone
• ↑Renal artery stenosis
• ↑Catecholamines
• ↑Endothelin

Hemodynamic Factors
• ↑End diastolic pressure
• ↑Afterload
• ↑Left ventricular stress
• ↑Myocardial length
• Ischemia

Electrolyte Abnormalities
• ↑Potassium
• ↑Magnesium
• Hyponatremia
• Alkalosis

Iatrogenic Factors
• Inotropes–tachycardia
• Vasodilators–hypotension
• Antiarrhythmics–proarrhythmia
• Diuretics–electrolytic abnormalities

Cardiac Arrhythmias
• Palpitations
• Syncope
• Orthostasis

Sudden Death
• Heart block
• Bradyarrhythmias
• Ventricular tachycardia
• Ventricular fibrillation
• Electromechanical dissociation

with electrolyte depletion and exposure to drugs with arrhythmogenic potential.

The benefits of maintaining sinus rhythm are outlined in **Table 6**.7. Atrial-ventricular synchrony improves ventricular filling and cardiac output, reduces risk of cardiogenic thromboemboli, and eliminates the need for some antiarrhythmic agents. Prognosis is improved when patients remain in normal sinus rhythm. When AF becomes chronic and refractory, atrial ventricular nodal ablation with implantation of a permanent rate-responsive ventricular pacemaker regularizes the rhythm, providing improved diastolic filling, as well as restoring an appropriate rate response to activity. This approach often results in substantial functional improvement as judged by NYHA-FC even with relatively severe LVD. Newer AF ablating techniques are also proving successful in selected patients with this arrhythmia. The surgical Maze procedure can be added to other cardiac procedures if indicated.

TABLE 6.7 — IMPORTANCE OF MAINTAINING SINUS RHYTHM IN HEART FAILURE

- Atrial-ventricular synchrony improves ventricular filling and cardiac output
- Reduces risk of cardiogenic thromboemboli
- Controlled rate response during exercise
- Eliminates need for some antiarrhythmics
- Attenuates tachycardia-induced heart failure
- Prognosis better
- Less symptoms

For patients at risk for ventricular arrhythmia and SCD, clinical data increasingly support implantation of an automatic cardioverter defibrillating device. In the hands of an experienced electrophysiologic team, this procedure carries very low morbidity and mortality and offers a significant degree of protection.

Comorbid Conditions

Table 6.8 lists important comorbidities that might be helpful to address when patients present with HF. Specific goals can be outlined for management of various comorbid conditions common in HF patients including:

- Diabetes
- Peripheral vascular disease
- Chronic obstructive pulmonary disease.

The importance of ensuring that a patient is euthyroid and the need for avoiding certain insulin-sensitizing compounds when the patient is congested have been discussed. Eliminating smoking, administration of flu and pneumonia vaccines, aggressive treatment of infectious bronchitis, and consideration of sleep apnea with treatment if appropriate, all can be helpful in patients with pulmonary difficulties. Patients with peripheral vascular disease should have aggressive risk factor management to attenuate progression. When degenerative joint disease is present, patients should avoid the regular use of NSAIDs, including the more recently developed COX-2 antagonists. Also important to these patients is maintaining body weight within 15% of predicted ideal.

Common Pitfalls

Table 6.9 lists some of the common pitfalls that complicate evaluation and treatment of HF.

Use of potentially harmful medications, such as Class 1 antiarrhythmic drugs and NSAIDs or insulin-sensitizing thiazolidinedione drugs may exacerbate clinical symptoms. Excessive intravascular volume depletion with diuretics can be counterproductive by producing orthostatic symptoms and further activating

TABLE 6.8 — APPROACH TO COMORBIDITIES

Comorbidity	Important Issue
Diabetes	• Maintain body weight within 15% of ideal • $HgbA_{1C} <7\%$ • On ACEI • Ensure euthyroid • Avoid thiazolidinedione compounds when patient congested
COPD	• Stop smoking • Live in smoke-free environment • Influenza/pneumonia vaccines • Aggressive treatment of infections • Consider sleep apnea studies and treat if appropriate • Bronchodilators if response demonstrated • Pulmonary rehabilitation • Chronic oxygen use
Peripheral vascular disease	• On aspirin, ACEI, statin • Interventional cardiology review of anatomy with revascularization if possible • Make sure left ventricular function quantified
Degenerative joint disease	• Avoid regular use of nonsteroidal anti-inflammatory agents • Maintain body weight within 15% of ideal • Exercise programs

Abbreviations: ACEI, angiotension-converting enzyme inhibitor; $HgbA_{1C}$, glycosylated hemoglobin A_{1C}; COPD, chronic obstructive pulmonary disease.

6

TABLE 6.9 — COMMON PITFALLS IN THE EVALUATION AND TREATMENT OF HEART FAILURE

- Improper syndrome recognition:
  - Symptoms actually unrelated or minimally related to cardiac dysfunction
  - Treatment begun late in the course of the illness
  - Failure to recognize presence of comorbidities
- Ignoring underlying disease state/comorbidities:
  - Not correcting areas of reversible myocardial ischemia
  - Not considering patients for standard (though higher risk) surgical procedures such as valve repair/replacement or left ventricular aneurysmectomy
  - Unrecognized hypothyroidism/hyperthyroidism
  - Poorly controlled diabetes mellitus
  - Inadequate control of hypertension
  - Not treating dyslipidemia
  - Not treating chronic obstructive pulmonary disease
  - Not considering possibility of cardiac metastasis in malignancies
- Not recognizing/treating certain comorbidities:
  - Intercurrent infections—bronchitis, pneumonia, cellulitis
  - Hypoventilation—sleep apnea syndromes
- Patient-related difficulties:
  - Poor compliance with drug treatment protocols
  - Inadequate salt and water restriction
  - Excessive alcohol consumption
  - Cigarette smoking/nicotine exposure
  - Obesity
  - Cardiovascular deconditioning
- Pharmacotherapeutic issues:
  - Inadequate ACEI therapy (or drug not begun)
  - Inadequate β-blocker therapy (or drug not begun)
  - Suboptimal doses of vasodilators
  - Ineffective diuretic prescription
  - Excessive diuresis
  - Discontinuation of digoxin in stable CHF patients

- Down-titration of ACEI instead of diuretics for hypotension or azotemia
- Concomitant use of potentially harmful medications (certain antiarrhythmics, nonsteroidal anti-inflammatory drugs, β-blockers or calcium channel antagonists in certain circumstances, and TZD insulin-sensitizing oral hypoglycemics)
• Other treatment concerns/pitfalls:
- Administration of anthracyclines
- Not evaluating/correcting/controlling atrial fibrillation
- Inappropriate drug treatment of certain ventricular arrhythmias
- Not considering pacemaker therapies for chronotropic incompetence and wide QRS
- Not preventing/treating hypokalemia, hypomagnesemia, hyponatremia
- Salt/fluid administration parenterally for orthostatic hypotension or hyponatremia
- Failure to use hemodynamic monitoring to resolve confusing or challenging situations

6

Abbreviations: ACEI, angiotensin-converting enzyme inhibitor; CHF, congestive heart failure; TZD, thiazolidinedione (rosiglitazone/pioglitazone).

neurohumoral factors important in the pathophysiology of HF. Inadequate ACEI doses or failure to start ACEI therapy is a major difficulty. Every attempt should be made to get patients to target ACEI doses. Rather than sacrificing the ACEI in an aggressively diuresed patient, the diuretic dose should be decreased. Orthostatic hypotension generally responds to reduction in diuretics or possibly vasodilators. When volume status is uncertain, hemodynamic monitoring resolves many dilemmas.

Although the list of pitfalls is extensive, it is not complete. Most of the perplexing problems in clinical practice can be solved by first carefully revisiting the history, physical examination, and diagnostic evaluation, and then obtaining a right-heart physiologic assessment. Although retracing the steps and updating diagnostic information may seem costly and time-consuming, this must be viewed in the context of the enormous problem of recurrent hospitalizations for inadequately or improperly treated patients. The average cost of a HF admission in the United States is (arguably) $7,000 to $14,000, and preventing two or three recurrent admissions will certainly justify the expense of a right-heart catheterization, a coronary angiogram, and a repeat echocardiogram or ambulatory monitor, as well as the time spent in revisiting the history and physical examination.

Summary

Figure 6.6 gives an integrated overview of HF therapeutics. In summary, the general approach to HF treatment outlined in this chapter requires a thorough diagnostic assessment, active treatment of ischemia and other cardiac derangements whenever possible, and a careful functional assessment of the individual patient. This should be followed by:

- Dietary and lifestyle modification
- Rehabilitation and activity counseling
- Family counseling
- Prescription of a rational therapeutic protocol
- Electrophysiologic evaluation
- Follow-up at regularly scheduled intervals.

FIGURE 6.6 — TAILORING HEART FAILURE THERAPIES

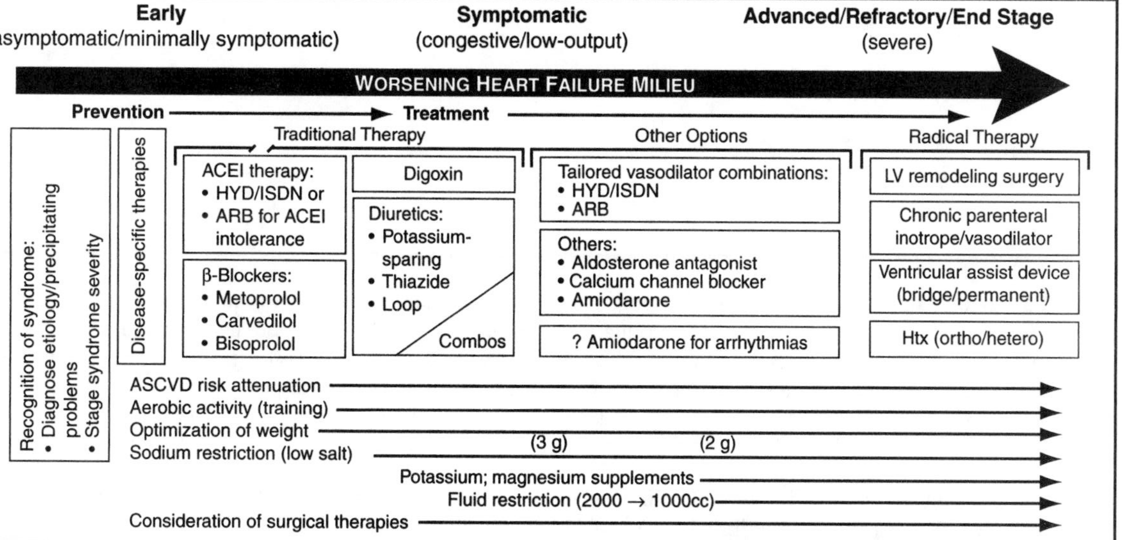

Early (asymptomatic/minimally symptomatic)	Symptomatic (congestive/low-output)	Advanced/Refractory/End Stage (severe)

WORSENING HEART FAILURE MILIEU

Prevention → Treatment

Traditional Therapy

	Treatment		
	Symptomatic	Other Options	Radical Therapy

ACEI therapy:
• HYD/ISDN or
• ARB for ACEI intolerance

β-Blockers:
• Metoprolol
• Carvedilol
• Bisoprolol

Digoxin

Diuretics:
• Potassium-sparing
• Thiazide
• Loop
Combos

Tailored vasodilator combinations:
• HYD/ISDN
• ARB

Others:
• Aldosterone antagonist
• Calcium channel blocker
• Amiodarone

? Amiodarone for arrhythmias

LV remodeling surgery

Chronic parenteral inotrope/vasodilator

Ventricular assist device (bridge/permanent)

Htx (ortho/hetero)

Disease-specific therapies

ASCVD risk attenuation
Aerobic activity (training)
Optimization of weight
Sodium restriction (low salt) ———————— (3 g) ———— (2 g)

Potassium; magnesium supplements
Fluid restriction (2000 → 1000cc)

Consideration of surgical therapies

Recognition of syndrome:
• Diagnose etiology/precipitating problems
• Stage syndrome severity

Continued

6

159

Abbreviations: ACEI, angiotensin-converting enzyme inhibitor; ARB, angiotensin receptor blocker; ASCVD, atherosclerotic cardiovascular disease; HF, heart failure; Htx, heart transplant; HYD/ISDN, hydralazine/isosorbide dinitrate; LV, left ventricle; ortho, orthotopic; hetero, heterotopic.

The approach to patients with HF is based on the fact that patients inevitably move from prevention to treatment strategies as they progress from insidious or asymptomatic HF due to left ventricular systolic dysfunction to symptomatic, severe and advanced, or refractory HF. At the core of HF management is disease-specific therapy as well as lifestyle modification. Drug treatment protocols that are particularly important include ACEIs, β-adrenergic blockers, ARBs, and aldosterone antagonists (spironolactone and eplerinone). If congestion is present, diuretics and digoxin are important agents.

7

Pharmacotherapeutics

Introduction

In Chapter 6, *General Treatment Approaches*, an overarching approach to heart failure (HF) therapy is presented. In this chapter, specific drugs used in patients with varying degrees of HF are discussed. Our approach is largely based on therapeutic algorithms tested in an HF disease-management program. They have been refined and edited based on clinical experience. The algorithms were initially created utilizing best evidence from clinical trials that have shaped clinical practice. These clinical trials (see Chapter 5, *Clinical Trials Shaping Heart Failure Therapeutics*) influenced the HF guidelines from the American College of Cardiology, the American Heart Association, the European Society of Cardiology, and the Heart Failure Society of America. We will specifically address use of angiotensin-converting enzyme inhibitors (ACEIs), diuretics, β-adrenergic blockers, digoxin, aldosterone antagonists, and angiotensin receptor blockers (ARBs). **Figure 7.1** summarizes, in schematic fashion, an overall pharmacologic approach to management of HF. Unfortunately, as addressed in Chapter 8, *Rational Polypharmacy* (Table 8.1), polypharmacy is common and necessary in HF patients to achieve the desired attenuation of morbidity and mortality.

After judging the severity of HF based on degree of dyspnea, fluid retention status, or hemodynamics, one should determine if clinically significant volume overload is present. If this is not the case, ACEIs should be initiated and titration to target doses begun. β-Blockers should subsequently be added to this proto-

FIGURE 7.1 — PHARMACOLOGIC MANAGEMENT OF HEART FAILURE

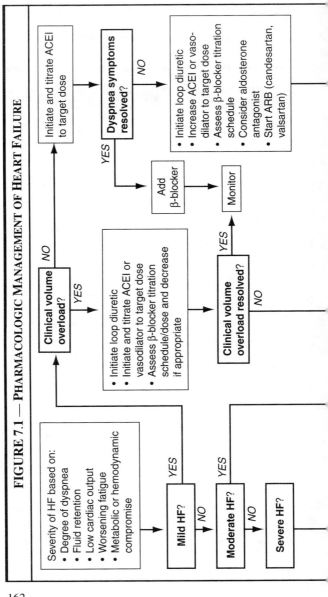

162

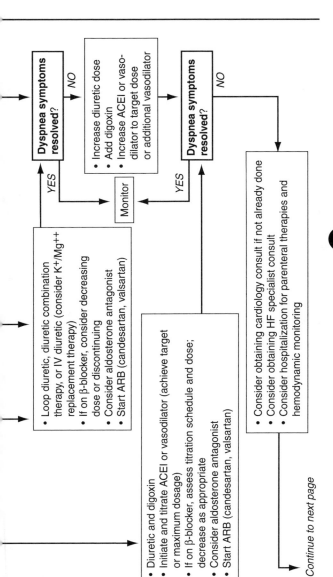

- Loop diuretic, diuretic combination therapy, or IV diuretic (consider K^+/Mg^{++} replacement therapy)
- If on β-blocker, consider decreasing dose or discontinuing
- Consider aldosterone antagonist
- Start ARB (candesartan, valsartan)

Dyspnea symptoms resolved?

YES

NO

- Increase diuretic dose
- Add digoxin
- Increase ACEI or vasodilator to target dose or additional vasodilator

Monitor

- Diuretic and digoxin
- Initiate and titrate ACEI or vasodilator (achieve target or maximum dosage)
- If on β-blocker, assess titration schedule and dose; decrease as appropriate
- Consider aldosterone antagonist
- Start ARB (candesartan, valsartan)

YES

Dyspnea symptoms resolved?

NO

- Consider obtaining cardiology consult if not already done
- Consider obtaining HF specialist consult
- Consider hospitalization for parenteral therapies and hemodynamic monitoring

Continue to next page

7

163

Continued from previous page

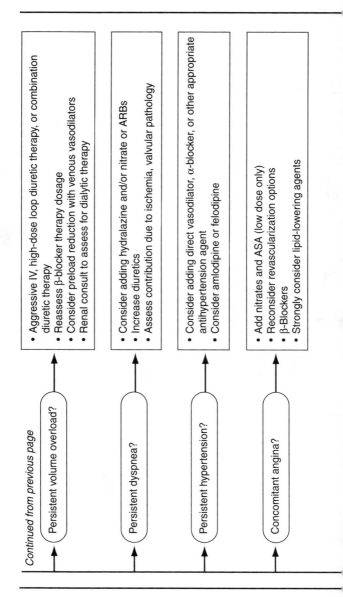

Persistent volume overload?
- Aggressive IV, high-dose loop diuretic therapy, or combination diuretic therapy
- Reassess β-blocker therapy dosage
- Consider preload reduction with venous vasodilators
- Renal consult to assess for dialytic therapy

Persistent dyspnea?
- Consider adding hydralazine and/or nitrate or ARBs
- Increase diuretics
- Assess contribution due to ischemia, valvular pathology

Persistent hypertension?
- Consider adding direct vasodilator, α-blocker, or other appropriate antihypertension agent
- Consider amlodipine or felodipine

Concomitant angina?
- Add nitrates and ASA (low dose only)
- Reconsider revascularization options
- β-Blockers
- Strongly consider lipid-lowering agents

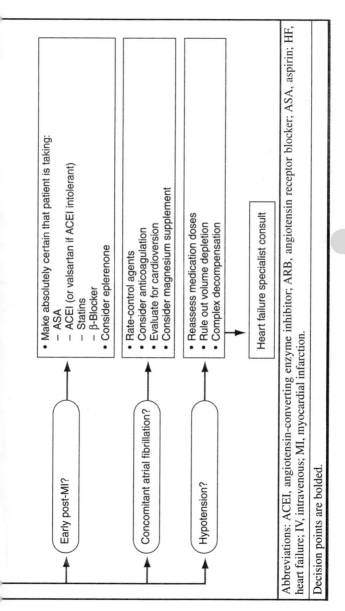

- Early post-MI?
  → • Make absolutely certain that patient is taking:
    - ASA
    - ACEI (or valsartan if ACEI intolerant)
    - Statins
    - β-Blocker
    - Consider eplerenone

- Concomitant atrial fibrillation?
  → • Rate-control agents
    • Consider anticoagulation
    • Evaluate for cardioversion
    • Consider magnesium supplement

- Hypotension?
  → • Reassess medication doses
    • Rule out volume depletion
    • Complex decompensation → Heart failure specialist consult

Abbreviations: ACEI, angiotensin-converting enzyme inhibitor; ARB, angiotensin receptor blocker; ASA, aspirin; HF, heart failure; IV, intravenous; MI, myocardial infarction.

Decision points are bolded.

165

col after optimization of ACEI dose has occurred. Depending upon the severity of congestion and hypotension, concomitant up-titration of ACEIs and β-blockers may be possible. In the patient without obvious volume overload but with significant symptoms of dyspnea, sometimes initiation of diuretics or increasing the diuretic dose is helpful, but right-heart catheterization might be warranted to more precisely determine filling pressures.[112,253] Usually, we turn to loop diuretics first. If the patient has presented with clinical volume overload, starting a loop diuretic with subsequent addition of an ACEI or an ARB (ie, candesartan or valsartan) in ACEI–intolerant patients may be preferable. Starting direct-acting vasodilators, such as a hydralazine (HYD)/isosorbide dinitrate (ISDN) combination, is a second option in this group.

The order of polypharmacy protocol is driven more by the historical development of these agents and approaches to their use. That is, clinical trials went from adding ACEIs, then β-blockers, then aldosterone antagonists, and now, ARBs. In all cases of HF with systolic left ventricular dysfunction (LVD), an attempt to initiate an ACEI is warranted. Perhaps the most challenging difficulty is balancing the need for diuresis in the patient with persistent clinical volume overload and borderline low blood pressure while up-titrating ACEI and β-blocker doses. As **Figure 7**.1 suggests, a variety of approaches can be taken. After establishing baseline therapy with diuretics, ACEIs (or alternative vasodilating drugs), and low doses of digoxin, other strategies can be pursued if difficulties persist; **Figure 7**.1 gives several suggestions that may be helpful. For persistent volume overload, intravenous (IV) loop diuretic therapy or combination loop/thiazide therapy may be helpful. Also, when persistent volume overload is present, one may consider down-titration or stopping β-blockers in certain circumstances. This may, however, be associated with increased adverse

166

events. Sometimes it is helpful to reduce preload with venous vasodilators (long-acting nitrate preparations). As the preload falls, the renal perfusion pressures sometimes improve, prompting more subsequent diuresis. A renal consultation for dialytic therapy may be a last option.

Persistent dyspnea sometimes responds to increasing diuretics when signs of congestion and volume overload are not present. In individuals with paroxysmal dyspnea and no evident congestion, one might consider ischemia or valvular pathology. Paroxysmal dyspnea is one of the classic angina surrogates in patients with active ischemia but no chest pain, particularly in diabetics. In individuals with persistent hypertension, one might consider adding HYD, ARBs, or a vasodilating calcium channel blocker (eg, amlodipine or felodipine) since clinical trials suggest no harm with these agents.

When angina pectoris is present in the HF setting, revascularization is the most critical strategy. Adding nitrates and aspirin to the patient's regimen can be important, as may reconsideration of the aggressiveness of the β-blocker prescription.

In patients with concomitant atrial fibrillation (AF), one must debate the pros and cons of rate control with pharmacologic or atrial ventricular nodal ablation strategies or rhythm control with electrical cardioversion, perhaps coupled with antiarrhythmic drugs. The pros and cons of these strategies will be subsequently reviewed.

When hypotension is present, one must determine the severity of the problem. Arguably, target blood pressure should be the lowest pressure with which a patient is not significantly symptomatic with orthostatic complaints and with which renal function is reasonably well maintained. When renal insufficiency occurs or the patient becomes orthostatic, one should reassess medications, doses, and administration strategies. Ruling out volume depletion is important. Backing

167

down the diuretic dose in a patient who is euvolemic or volume depleted is preferable to reducing ACEIs or β-blockers.

Most of the practical therapeutic suggestions that follow are specifically focused on patients with congestive heart failure (CHF) and low ejection fraction (EF). There is limited information available about the best tactics to pursue in those with CHF and so-called "preserved" LV function (sometimes referred to as diastolic HF or dysfunction). No trial to date has demonstrated the ability of a drug to decrease mortality in CHF when the left ventricular ejection fraction (LVEF) is >40%. Only one large scale trial has been done specifically in this group—the CHARM-Preserved trial (see Chapter 5, *Clinical Trials Shaping Heart Failure Therapeutics*). In this trial, 3025 patients were randomized to candesartan or placebo in addition to ACEIs in almost 20%, β-blockers in 56%, digoxin in 28%, calcium channel blockers in 31%, and diuretics in about 75%.[321] Over a median follow-up of 36.6 months, there was a significant reduction in HF hospitalizations, but no impact on mortality. The only other large clinical trial cohort was a subset of DIG trial subjects with CHF and preserved LV systolic function.[84] In that study, digoxin produced similar benefits: reduction in number of patients hospitalized for HF treatment but no impact on mortality. Thus only digoxin and candesartan have, to date, been demonstrated effective agents to reduce a morbidity end point in CHF patients with more normal LVEF.

Diuretics

Table 7.1 focuses on diuretics commonly used in patients with HF. Diuretics are reserved for congestive states, perhaps with the exception of spironolactone. Before instituting diuretic therapy, patients should be counseled on the importance of salt and water restriction. If a reasonable salt and water restriction is not imposed, diuretic therapy will often provoke severe electrolyte disturbances, particularly worsening hyponatremia. Diuretics should not be given on a regular daily basis until patients are well into New York Heart Association functional class (NYHA-FC) III CHF. Patients should be taught to monitor daily weight at home and adjust diuretic therapy as needed, omitting diuretics whenever possible to minimize side effects.

As HF advances, daily diuretics or even twice-daily diuretic therapy, generally with a loop diuretic, will be necessary. When loop diuretics are begun, potassium and magnesium repletion either with dietary adjustments or dietary supplements is critical. Often, using an aldosterone antagonist will help prevent hypokalemia. One or 2 diuretic-free days a week, even with relatively advanced HF, often eliminate electrolyte abnormalities. As **Table 7**.1 demonstrates, diuretic classes include:

- Thiazides
- Thiazide-related agents
- Loop diuretics
- Potassium-sparing diuretics.

Figure 7.2 presents a diuretic therapy algorithm based on signs and symptoms of volume overload. This strategy has proved particularly useful in more severely congested NYHA-FC III/IV patients and can be used in an outpatient setting with nurse phone-call follow-up.

Table 7.2 summarizes additional issues that are important when initiating diuretic therapy. As indicated, focus must be on the congested patient with consideration of pulsed or intermittent therapy. Elderly patients may require lower doses, and it is reasonable to start with the lowest effective dose of either a thiazide or a loop diuretic. If refractory congestion is present, a combination of a loop and a thiazide diuretic will ef-

TABLE 7.1 — MEDICATIONS COMMONLY USED FOR HEART FAILURE: DIURETICS

Generic (Trade) Drug	Initial Dose (mg)	Target Dose (mg)	Maximum Dose (mg)	Major Adverse Reactions
IV Diuretics				
Bumetanide (Bumex)	0.5 qd	As needed	10 qd	Postural hypotension; hypokalemia; hyponatremia; hyperglycemia; hypomagnesia; rash; rare severe reactions include pancreatitis, bone marrow suppression, and anaphylaxis
Chlorothiazide (Diuril)	250 bolus		1000 bid	
Ethacrynic acid (Edecrin)	50 qd		100 bid	
Furosemide (Lasix)	10-40 bolus/ (5-40 mg/h continuous infusion)		480/qd	
Torsemide (Demadex)	10 qd		200 qd	
Loop Diuretics				
Bumetanide (Bumex)	0.5-1.0 qd	As needed	10 qd	*Same as IV diuretics*
Ethacrynic acid (Edecrin)	50 qd		200 bid	
Furosemide (Lasix)	20-80 qd		240 bid	
Torsemide (Demadex)	10 qd		200 qd	

Potassium-Sparing Diuretics				
Amiloride (Midamor)	5 qd	As needed	20 qd	Little information for use in heart failure
Triamterene (Maxzide)	50 qd		100 bid	Little information for use in heart failure
Thiazide Diuretics				
Chlorthalidone (Hygroton)	25 qd	As needed	50 mg	*Same as IV diuretics*
Hydrochlorothiazide (HydroDIURIL)	25 qd		50 qd	
Thiazide-Related Diuretics				
Metolazone (Zaroxolyn)	2.5 qd	As needed	10 qd	*Same as IV diuretics;* hyponatremia/hypokalemia can be severe
Abbreviation: ACEI, angiotensin-converting enzyme inhibitor.				

FIGURE 7.2 — HEART FAILURE MANAGEMENT: DIURETIC THERAPY ALGORITHM

Heart failure? → **YES**

- NYHA Functional Class I/II patients may NOT require a regular diuretic regimen, especially if following sodium and fluid restriction recommendations and no signs of volume overload
- NYHA Functional Class III/IV patients usually require regular diuretic regimen

Clinical signs of increased filling pressure (volume overload) in a patient receiving maintenance diuretic therapy

Individualize diuretic therapy based on signs and symptoms of increased filling pressure:

Signs
- Jugular venous distention
- Tachycardia
- S_3 gallop
- Rales
- Abnormal abdominojugular reflux
- Edema (peripheral, ascites, or anasarca)

Radiographic fluid redistribution, pulmonary edema, or pleural effusion

Symptoms
- Dyspnea, orthopnea, paroxysmal nocturnal dyspnea
- History of weight gain >3 lb within 24 h to 1 wk

If mild volume overload (3- to 5-lb weight gain and other signs/symptoms)

Furosemide (or equivalent) Oral Dose		
<120 mg/d	≥120 mg/d, kidney function normal	≥120 mg/d, serum creatinine >2.5 mg/dL
Double oral furosemide AM dose and potassium supplement × 1 d	Add metolazone 2.5 mg and double potassium supplement × 1 d	Add metolazone 5 mg and double potassium supplement × 1 d

Reassess via telephone or outpatient-department visits

If weight gain or symptoms persist, **continue same plan as above × 1-3 d**

Reassess via telephone or outpatient-department visits

If Assessment Remains Unchanged	
Furosemide (or equivalent) Oral Dose <120 mg/d	Furosemide (or equivalent) Oral Dose ≥120 mg/d
Increase dose to 1.5 × previous daily dose (eg, was taking 80 mg q AM, increase to 120 mg q AM or was taking 40 mg bid, increase to 60 mg bid)	Administer IV furosemide (or equivalent) equal to AM oral dose and continue doubled potassium supplement × 1 d

Continued to next page

173

Reassess via telephone or outpatient-department visits

If weight gain or symptoms persist and assessment does not improve, **Notify Physician.**

If Moderate-Severe Overload (eg, >5-lb weight gain and other signs/symptoms)

Furosemide (or equivalent) Oral Dose <120 mg/d	Furosemide (or equivalent) Oral Dose ≥120 mg/d
• Add metolazone 2.5 mg (5 mg if renal insufficiency [serum creatinine >2.5 mg/dL]) 30 minutes before furosemide qd × 2 d • Double potassium supplement × 3 d • Double oral furosemide AM dose × 2 d	• Add metolazone 2.5 mg (5 mg if renal insufficiency)* 30 minutes before furosemide qd × 2 d • Double potassium supplement × 3 d • Administer IV furosemide equal to AM oral dose × 2 d

* Option: Instead of metolazone, add chlorothiazide (Diuril) 250 mg IV (500 mg if renal insufficiency/failure) 30 minutes before furosemide qd × 2 d

Obtain serum potassium level within 3 to 7 d after aggressive diuretic administration

NOTE:	1. Monitor potassium level. If it remains low despite potassium supplements, check magnesium level. Refer to **Table 7.5** for additional potassium and/or magnesium dosing information.
	2. If serum potassium level is >5.0 mEq/L, do not administer additional potassium as noted. Obtain serum potassium level within 48 h of aggressive diuretic administration.

Reassess patient appropriately and if symptoms persist, **Notify Physician.**

Abbreviation: NYHA-FC, New York Heart Association functional class.

TABLE 7.2 — ISSUES TO CONSIDER WHEN INITIATING DIURETIC THERAPY

- Focus on the congested patient
- Consider pulsed or intermittent diuretic therapy
- Elderly patients require lower doses
- Start with lowest effective dose
- Combine different classes for added diuretic effect
- Monitoring and therapy for magnesium <1.8 mg/dL, potassium <3.5 or >5.0 mEq/dL, sodium <135 mEq/dL, creatinine >3.0 mg/dL
- Couple with sodium and free-water restriction
- Watch for hyponatremia
- Rapid diuresis may require electrolyte replenishment
- May be able to stop diuretics in stable noncongested patients

7

fect better diuresis. Monitoring for electrolyte abnormalities is extremely important, as is sodium and free-water restriction. Excessive sodium intake is the most significant factor in producing hypokalemia in the setting of thiazide and loop diuretic use. Hyponatremia will occur with vigorous diuretic therapy unless free-water intake is restricted. Rapid diuresis will usually require electrolyte replenishment. Diuretics should be stopped in stable, noncongestive patients.

Common problems seen with diuretics are listed in **Table 7.3** and include the electrolyte disturbances already alluded to, as well as hyperglycemia, insulin resistance, decreased insulin secretion, and predisposition to nonketotic hyperosmolar states. Diuretics also precipitate lipid abnormalities, including increased low-density lipoprotein, very low-density lipoprotein, total cholesterol, and triglyceride levels. Several toxicities related singularly to specific agents can be noted. Furosemide (Lasix) and ethacrynic acid (Edecrin) can produce ototoxicity. Acetazolamide (Diamox) can produce metabolic acidosis, and the potassium-sparing diuretics obviously can be associated with hyperkalemia.

TABLE 7.3 — COMMON PROBLEMS WITH DIURETICS

Electrolyte Disturbances
- Hyponatremia
- Hypokalemia (hyperkalemia with potassium-sparing agents)
- Hypomagnesemia
- Hypocalciuria
- Hyperurecemia
- Metabolic alkalosis

Carbohydrate Metabolism Perturbation
- Hyperglycemia
- Insulin resistance
- Decreased insulin secretion
- Nonketotic hyperosmoler state

Lipid Abnormalities
- Increased low-density lipoprotein
- Increased very low-density lipoprotein
- Increased total cholesterol
- Increased triglycerides

Diuretic-Specific Side Effects
- Furosemide and ethacrynic acid*—ototoxicity
- Acetazolamide—metabolic acidosis
- Potassium-sparing diuretics—generally, hyperkalemia

* Ethacrynic acid is highly ototoxic and should only be used in patients allergic (sulfa allergies) to other loop diuretics.

Table 7.4 compares the various loop diuretic agents, illustrating that bioavailability is widely varied. Bumetanide (Bumex) and torsemide (Demadex) are far more bioavailable than furosemide. Some believe, therefore, that bumetanide and torsemide might be better agents to use in severely volume-overloaded patients who are experiencing mesenteric congestion and have difficulties with drug absorption from the outset. Others argue that by simply increasing the dose of furosemide, one alleviates the problem of reduced

TABLE 7.4 — RELATIVE DOSES: LOOP DIURETICS			
Diuretic	**Bioavailability (%)**	**IV-to-Oral Conversion**	**Relative Potency (mg)**
Bumetanide	75	1:1	1
Ethacrynic acid	100	1:1	50
Furosemide	50	1:2	40
Torsemide	80	1:1	20
Abbreviation: IV, intravenous.			

bioavailability. With the more bioavailable agents, IV-to-oral drug conversion is generally about 1:1. Furosemide, on the other hand, has a 1:2 IV-to-oral dose conversion ratio.

Table 7.5 is a potassium and magnesium supplement algorithm. Because loop and thiazide diuretics waste both of these cations, it is important to monitor potassium and magnesium levels to determine points at which repletion should be begun or intensified. However, serum magnesium levels may not reflect total-body magnesium depletion. Magnesium supplementation can be helpful in maintaining appropriate serum potassium levels.

Aldosterone Antagonists

Figure 7.3 reviews the important new tactic of prescribing the aldosterone antagonists eplerenone (Inspra) and spironolactone (Aldactone). These drugs may be added as an adjunctive neurohormonal blocking agent in patients who are stable on otherwise appropriate HF therapy. Spironolactone has been studied in CHF generally and eplerenone in an acutely post–myocardial infarction (MI) HF cohort.

Dosing information on the aldosterone antagonists is presented in **Table 7.6**.

TABLE 7.5 — HEART FAILURE MANAGEMENT: POTASSIUM AND MAGNESIUM ORAL-DOSE THERAPY

Level (mEq/dL)	POTASSIUM*			Recheck Potassium
	Serum Creatinine Level			
	≤1.5 mg/dL	>1.5 to ≤2.5 mg/dL	>2.5 mg/dL	
>5.5	Notify physician			Per physician order
5.1 to 5.5	↓ Dose 20 mEq qd	↓ Dose 20-40 mEq qd		5 d to 1 wk
4.0 to 5.0	No intervention			As needed
3.7 to 3.9	40 mEq	30 mEq	20 mEq	Next day to 1 wk
3.4 to 3.6	40 mEq × 2 doses	40 mEq + 20 mEq	40 mEq	Next day†
3.0 to 3.3	40 mEq × 3 doses	40 mEq × 2 doses	40 mEq + 20 mEq	
<3.0 *Notify physician*	40 mEq × 4 doses	40 mEq × 3 doses	40 mEq × 2 doses	Next morning†

MAGNESIUM			
Level (mg/dL)	Serum Creatinine Level		Recheck Magnesium
	≤2.5 mg/dL	>2.5 mg/dL	
>3.0‡	Notify physician		Per physician order
2.5 to 3.0	↓ Dose by 1/2; if not on supplement, notify physician		1 wk
2.0 to 2.5	No intervention		As needed
1.9	Uro-mag 140 mg × 2	Uro-mag 140 mg × 1	24 h to 1 wk after last dose
1.3 to 1.8	Uro-mag 280 mg × 4§	Uro-mag 280 mg × 2§	24-48 h after last dose
≤1.2‡	Uro-mag 560 mg × 4§	Uro-mag 560 mg × 2§	24 h after last dose

* Parenteral potassium replenishment may be considered preferable in NPO patients or in urgent situations where cardiac or neurologic symptoms are related to hypokalemia.
† If potassium continues to remain <3.5 mEq/L at recheck: order magnesium level (in addition to giving more potassium per nomogram).
‡ Obtain electrocardiogram to evaluate QT interval. If QT interval is >0.56 sec, notify physician.
§ Space doses throughout the day; may cause diarrhea.

7

FIGURE 7.3 — HEART FAILURE MANAGEMENT: ALDOSTERONE ANTAGONIST ALGORITHM

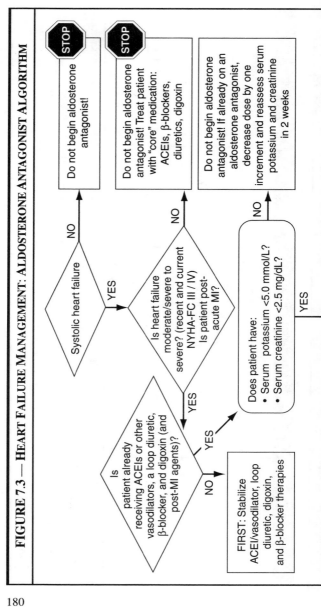

Systolic heart failure

NO → Do not begin aldosterone antagonist!

YES ↓

Is patient already receiving ACEIs or other vasodilators, a loop diuretic, β-blocker, and digoxin (and post-MI agents)?

NO → FIRST: Stabilize ACEI/vasodilator, loop diuretic, digoxin, and β-blocker therapies

YES ↓

Is heart failure moderate/severe to severe? (recent and current NYHA-FC III / IV) Is patient post-acute MI?

NO → STOP Do not begin aldosterone antagonist! Treat patient with "core" medication: ACEIs, β-blockers, diuretics, digoxin

YES ↓

Does patient have:
• Serum potassium <5.0 mmol/L?
• Serum creatinine <2.5 mg/dL?

NO → Do not begin aldosterone antagonist! If already on an aldosterone antagonist, decrease dose by one increment and reassess serum potassium and creatinine in 2 weeks

YES

Spironolactone was studied in CHF generally and eplerenone acutely post-MI.
- Begin spironolactone at 12.5-mg daily and increase to 25-mg daily
- Begin eplerenone at 25-mg daily and increase to 50-mg daily
- Consider decreasing dose of supplemental potassium and other diuretic medications
- Monitor serum potassium level within 5 to 7 days, at one month, and periodically thereafter, especially after any change in dose or in the case of concomitant medications that affect potassium balance (ACEIs or angiotensin receptor blocker therapies)

If dose is NOT tolerated due to hyperkalemia, follow incremental/decremental dose schedule below until serum lab work goals of potassium <5.0 mmol/L and creatinine <2.5 mg are achieved, and adjust other medications that contribute to hyperkalemia

Aldosterone Antagonist Incremental/Decremental Dose Schedule

	Maximum Dose	Standard Dose	Decreasing Increments	
Spironolactone (Aldactone)	50 mg qd	12.5-25 mg qd	12.5 mg qd or 25 mg qod	Discontinue
Eplerenone (Inspra)	50 mg qd	25-50 mg qd	25 qod	Discontinue

NOTE: Men may experience gynecomastia or breast pain with spironolactone, which may require discontinuation of therapy.

Abbreviations: ACEI, angiotensin-converting enzyme inhibitor; CHF, congestive heart failure; MI, myocardial infarction; NYHA-FC, New York Heart Association functional class.

| | | | TABLE 7.6 — MEDICATIONS COMMONLY USED IN HEART FAILURE: ALDOSTERONE ANTAGONISTS | | |

Generic (Trade) Drug	Initial Dose (mg)	Target Dose (mg)	Maximum Dose (mg)	Major Adverse Reactions
Eplerenone (Inspra)	25 qd	50 qd	50 qd	Similar to spironolactone without gynecomastia, less hyperkalemia
Spironolactone (Aldactone)	25 qd	As needed	100 bid as diuretic	Hypotension, especially if administered with ACEI; rash; gynecomastia; hyper-kalemia

Spironolactone prescribed in usual doses (12.5 to 25 mg qd) in symptomatic CHF patients is generally nondiuretic but associated with reduced morbidity and mortality, as is eplerenone when used in the post-MI HF population as described below.

The principal risk of eplerenone and spironolactone is hyperkalemia. Spironolactone is associated with painful gynecomastia (not seen with eplerenone) that often requires discontinuation of therapy.

Low-dose spironolactone (ie, 12.5 and 25 mg qd) did not provoke serious problems with hyperkalemia in most participants in RALES. The same can be said for eplerenone as demonstrated in EPHESUS. It is important to note that 100% of the patients in the RALES trial were on loop diuretics, which may account for the low incidence of hyperkalemia. The EPHESUS study design did not require diuretic use, but rather ACE and β-blocker therapy. Nonetheless, hyperkalemia can be seen with eplerenone and spironolactone. One must monitor patients carefully to prevent this potentially devastating difficulty. Serum potassium should be checked within 5 to 7 days of initiating therapy, at 1 month, and periodically thereafter. Spironolactone and eplerenone in these doses do not confer benefit by inducing additive diuresis. Rather, they are likely working solely by neurohormonal blocking activity. Higher doses of spironolactone may effect an increased diuresis. Anti-aldosterone doses of spironolactone for heart failure should not exceed 50 mg daily. The maximum dose for eplerenone is 50 mg daily.

Angiotensin-Converting Enzyme Inhibitors

A theme throughout this text has been the extraordinary importance of ACEIs in patients with systolic LVD and HF. Reemphasizing this fact are **Figure 7.4** and **Figure 7.5**. **Figure 7.4** summarizes large mor-

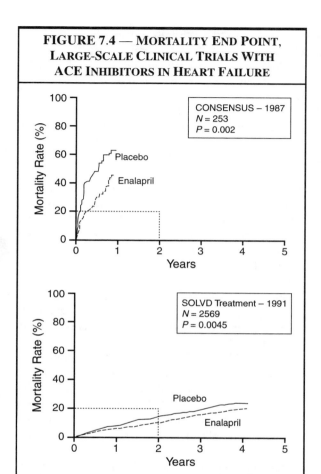

FIGURE 7.4 — MORTALITY END POINT, LARGE-SCALE CLINICAL TRIALS WITH ACE INHIBITORS IN HEART FAILURE

CONSENSUS – 1987
$N = 253$
$P = 0.002$

SOLVD Treatment – 1991
$N = 2569$
$P = 0.0045$

tality end-point clinical trials with ACEIs in HF demonstrating the consistent reduction in mortality seen in a wide spectrum of HF populations. **Figure 7.5** focuses on four major mortality end-point clinical trials with ACEIs in HF and LVD post-MI. **Table 7.7** summarizes the commonly used ACEIs in these patients. Arguably, the effects of ACEIs in HF patients are drug-class specific. However, not all ACEIs have been stud-

184

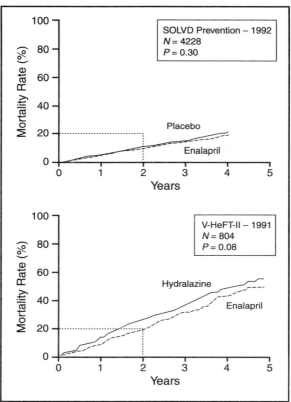

Abbreviations: CONSENSUS, Cooperative North Scandinavian Enalapril Survival Study; SOLVD, Studies of Left Ventricular Dysfunction (treatment and prevention arms); V-HeFT-II, Vasodilator-Heart Failure Trial II.

Heart failure mortality end point trials with curves normalized to years of follow-up and mortality rates so that the vagaries of the different patient populations (mortality of placebo group) and magnitude of treatment effects can be compared from trial to trial. Curves are similarly constructed in **Figures 7.5** and **7.6**.

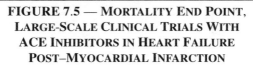

FIGURE 7.5 — MORTALITY END POINT, LARGE-SCALE CLINICAL TRIALS WITH ACE INHIBITORS IN HEART FAILURE POST–MYOCARDIAL INFARCTION

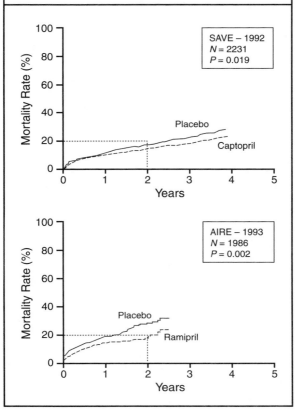

ied in HF populations, and benazepril (Lotensin) and moexipril (Univasc) do not carry Food and Drug Administration labeling approbation for HF therapy.

We favor using agents studied in HF so that the target doses demonstrated effective can become the goal. Target doses, for example, are 10 mg bid for

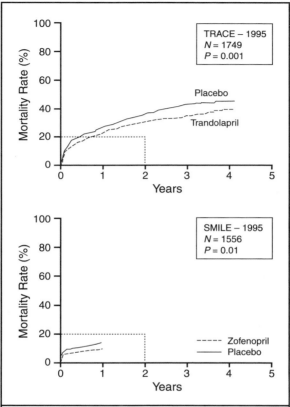

Abbreviations: ACE, angiotensin-converting enzyme; AIRE, Acute Infarction Ramipril Efficacy [study]; SAVE, Survival and Ventricular Enlargement; SMILE, Survival of Myocardial Infarction: Long-Term Evaluation; TRACE, Trandolapril Cardiac Evaluation [study].

enalapril (Vasotec) and 50 mg tid for captopril (Capoten). Oftentimes, it is tempting not to optimize dose because of fear of hypotension, renal insufficiency, or hyperkalemia. Although these concerns may be reasonable, in most patients the dose can be effectively up-

TABLE 7.7 — MEDICATIONS COMMONLY USED FOR HEART FAILURE: ACE INHIBITORS

Generic (Trade) Drug	Initial Dose (mg)	Target Dose (mg)	Maximum Dose (mg)	Major Adverse Reactions
Benazepril (Lotensin)*	2.5 or 5 bid	20 bid	20 bid	Hypotension, hyperkalemia, renal insufficiency, cough, skin rash, angioedema, neutropenia
Captopril (Capoten)	6.25-12.5 tid	50 tid	100 tid	
Enalapril (Vasotec)	2.5 bid	10 bid	20 bid	
Fosinopril (Monopril)	2.5 or 5 bid	20 bid	20 bid	
Lisinopril (Prinivil, Zestril)	5 qd	20 qd	40 qd	
Moexipril (Univasc)*	7.5 qd	30 qd	30 qd	
Quinapril (Accupril)	5 bid	20 bid	20 bid	
Ramipril (Altace)†	1.25 bid	10 qd	20 qd	
Trandolapril (Mavik)†	1.0 qd	4 qd	4 qd	

Abbreviation: ACE, angiotensin-converting enzyme.

* *Not* Food and Drug Administration (FDA)-labeled for heart failure therapy.
† FDA-labeled for heart failure therapy following acute myocardial infarction.

titrated to target dose if it is done carefully and with appropriate adjustments of other medications.

Table 7.8 specifically outlines several pitfalls that can be encountered during ACEI therapy for HF. Hypotension is a concern, however, and one can often decrease diuretic doses if patients are euvolemic and stop or reduce other vasodilators, particularly long-acting nitrates, to allow the blood pressure to rise. When worsening renal function follows initiation of ACEI therapy, one should make certain that the patient is not over-diuresed and has a reasonable blood pressure (>80 or 90 mm Hg systolic, but some require a blood pressure >100 mm Hg). Also, the clinician should make sure that nonsteroidal anti-inflammatory drugs have been stopped. If the blood urea nitrogen (BUN) and/or creatinine levels increase by <50%, maintaining the dose of ACEI is reasonable. If these values increase by >50%, we generally reduce the ACEI dose by one half. If the renal function measures increase by >100%, consider switching to an ARB or HYD/ISDN combination.

If hyperkalemia occurs, defined as serum potassium >5.5 mEq/dL, one should stop potassium-sparing diuretics and potassium supplements. If concomitant ARBs are being used, those agents should be stopped as well. Finally, decreasing or discontinuing the ACEI may be necessary. Perhaps the most irritating problem with ACEIs is cough. One must make certain that the cough is due to ACEI therapy rather than occult CHF or chronic obstructive pulmonary disease. Stop the ACEI only if the problem is intolerable, and when that is done, switch to an ARB (candesartan or valsartan).

β-Blockers

Figure 7.6 presents mortality curves from the four major clinical trials of β-blockers that demonstrated efficacy in a wide spectrum of patient popula-

TABLE 7.8 — PITFALLS OF ACE INHIBITOR THERAPY

Problem	Response
Hypotension	• Decrease diuretic dose if patient is euvolemic • Stop or decrease dose of other vasodilators (particularly long-acting nitrates) • Down-titrate dose of ACEI
Worsening renal function	• Make sure patient not overdiuresed • Make sure patient has reasonable blood pressure • Make sure NSAID is stopped • If BUN/creatinine increased by <50%, maintain therapy • If BUN/creatinine increased by >50%, reduce ACEI dose by 50% • Discontinue non–ACEI vasodilators • If BUN/creatinine increase >100%, switch to ARB or HYD/ISDN combination
Hyperkalemia	• Stop potassium-sparing diuretics • Stop potassium supplements • Stop concomitant ARB • Decrease ACE inhibitor dose
Cough	• Make sure cough is ACE inhibitor related • Stop ACEI only if problem is intolerable • Consider alternative vasodilators like HYD/ISDN or ARB

Abbreviations: ACEI, angiotensin-converting enzyme inhibitor; ARB, angiotensin receptor blocker; BUN, blood urea nitrogen; HYD, hydralazine; ISDN, isosorbide dinitrate; NSAID, nonsteroidal anti-flammatory drug.

tions. Carvedilol (Coreg), bisoprolol (Zebeta), and long-acting metoprolol (Toprol-XL) have all lowered mortality conclusively in patients with mild to severe HF. **Table 7.9** lists the β-blockers important to consider in HF settings. β-Adrenergic blockade should not be instituted until patients are stable on an appropriate baseline medication protocol, which includes an ACEI or alternative vasodilating agent in near-target doses.[32,40,156] β–Blockade must be begun with low doses and titrated slowly, over weeks or months, to target doses.

Table 7.10 emphasizes important issues regarding β-blocker therapy in HF. First, one should prescribe these drugs for every patient who has recently suffered a Q-wave MI. The CAPRICORN trial suggested that even in the thrombolytic and ACEI era, carvedilol can provide substantial mortality reduction in post-MI patients with reduced EFs.[50] Experience has taught us that β-blockers are best initiated when patients are not significantly congested, and one should avoid treating NYHA-FC IV patients with β-blockers unless they have been diuresed adequately.

Nonselective β-blockers with vasodilating properties (eg, carvedilol) may be preferred in some patients, but definitive evidence is yet to come. COMET compared carvedilol with lower-dose short-acting metoprolol in a wide range of HF patients.[21,22,88,108,238,261] In that trial, carvedilol reduced HF morbidity and mortality significantly more than the short-acting metoprolol preparation. No similar data comparing long-acting metoprolol with carvedilol are available (see comments in Chapter 5, *Clinical Trials Shaping Heart Failure Therapeutics*). Currently, carvedilol and long-acting metoprolol are the only FDA-approved β-blockers for use in HF patients. Some clinicians believe that long-acting metoprolol, a β_1-selective agent, may be better tolerated in patients with reactive airway disease. Others argue on the ba-

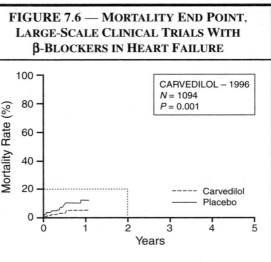

FIGURE 7.6 — MORTALITY END POINT, LARGE-SCALE CLINICAL TRIALS WITH β-BLOCKERS IN HEART FAILURE

CARVEDILOL – 1996
N = 1094
P = 0.001

Carvedilol
Placebo

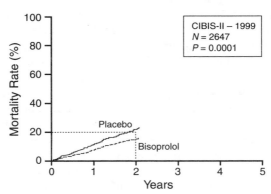

CIBIS-II – 1999
N = 2647
P = 0.0001

Placebo

Bisoprolol

sis of the COMET data that it is best to use a nonselective β-blocker in HF patients. Patients may initially deteriorate when β-blockers are begun (more congestion, weakness, and fatigue), but long term, patients generally improve, some dramatically.

Table 7.11 further explores the issue of β-blocker characteristics. First-generation drugs such as propranolol, timolol, pindolol, nadolol, and sotalol, are nonselec-

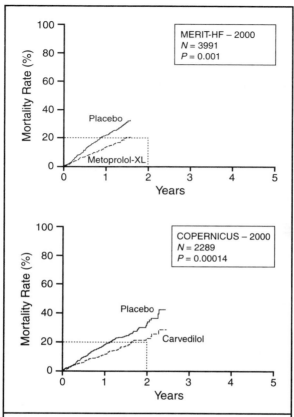

Abbreviations: CARVEDILOL, Effect of Carvedilol on Morbidity and Mortality in Patients With Chronic Heart Failure [trial]; CIBIS-II, Cardiac Insufficiency Bisoprolol Study-II; COPERNICUS, Carvedilol Prospective Randomized Cumulative Survival [trial]; MERIT-HF, Metoprolol CR/XL Randomized Intervention Trial in Heart Failure.

tive and nonvasodilating agents. Second-generation agents, such as atenolol, bisoprolol, and metoprolol, are β_1-receptor site selective, but are also nonvasodilating. Third-generation β-blocking agents, including bucindolol and carvedilol, are nonselective β_1 blockers and have

TABLE 7.9 — MEDICATIONS COMMONLY USED FOR HEART FAILURE: β-BLOCKERS

Generic (Trade) Drug	Initial Dose (mg)	Target Dose (mg)	Maximum Dose (mg)	Major Adverse Reactions
Bisoprolol (Zebeta)*	1.25 bid	5 qd (≤85 kg) 10 qd (>85 kg)	20 qd	Same as carvedilol (plus vivid dreams)
Carvedilol (Coreg)†	3.125 bid	25 bid (≤85 kg) 50 bid (>85 kg) (minimally effective dose 6.25 bid)	25 bid (≤85 kg) 50 bid (>85 kg)	Bradycardia, hypotension, atrioventricular block, worsening congestive heart failure, bronchospasm, fatigue
Metoprolol tartrate (Lopressor)*	12-25 bid	50 bid	100 bid	Same as carvedilol (may be somewhat better tolerated in patients with reactive airway disease)
Metoprolol succinate (Toprol-XL)‡	12-25 qd	200 qd	200 qd	

* Not Food and Drug Administration (FDA) labeled for heart failure therapy
† FDA approved for use in treating mild-to-severe heart failure.
‡ FDA approved for use in treating mild-to-moderate stable congestive heart failure.

TABLE 7.10 — β-BLOCKERS: ISSUES TO CONSIDER

- Prescribe in every post–myocardial infarction patient
- Start when patient not significantly congested
- Wait to prescribe for NYHA-FC IV patients until "dry"
- Based on COMET, short-acting metoprolol appears to be less effective
- Carvedilol (Coreg) and long-acting metoprolol (Toprol-XL) are currently the only FDA-approved agents for heart failure and should be β-blocker of choice
- Long-acting metoprolol may be better tolerated in patients with reactive airway disease (β_1-selective agent)
- Start with low dose and titrate slowly to target dose over many weeks (carvedilol 3.125 mg bid to 25 mg bid; long-acting metoprolol 12.5 mg qd to 200 mg qd)
- Short-term patients many deteriorate with more congestion, weakness, and fatigue, but long-term patients generally improve
- If a patient does not tolerate one agent, try the other

Abbreviations: COMET, Carvedilol or Metoprolol European Trial; FDA, Food and Drug Administration; NYHA-FC, New York Heart Association functional class.

vasodilating properties. Carvedilol also has α-adrenergic blocking effects, and this agent, therefore, produces the most complete blockade of myocyte cell surface adrenergic receptors.

Table 7.12 recapitulates the large-scale, mortality end point β-blocker trials in HF. These trials include the BEST study with bucindolol compared with placebo, which found a neutral effect in NYHA-FC III/IV CHF patients.[31] Perhaps this lack of beneficial effect was due to the fact that there were more minorities, more women, and more severe HF patients in this trial. The CAPRICORN trial compared carvedilol with placebo on a background of best medical therapies for acute MI

TABLE 7.11 — β-BLOCKERS IN HEART FAILURE	
Generation/Drugs	**Feature**
First Generation	
Carteolol	Nonselective, nonvasodilating
Nadolol	
Oxprenolol	
Penbutolol	
Pindolol	
Propranolol	
Sotalol	
Timolol	
Second Generation	
Atenolol	β_1-Selective, nonvasodilating
Betaxolol	
Bisoprolol	
Metoprolol	
Talinolol	
Acebutolol	β_1-Selective, vasodilating
Celiprolol	
Nebivolol	
Xamoterol	
Third Generation	
Bucindolol	Nonselective, vasodilating
Carvedilol	

patients with EFs <40%.[50] A 23% mortality reduction was noted despite modern-era post-MI therapies.

The COPERNICUS trial compared carvedilol with placebo in the most severely ill HF patient population yet studied with a β-blocker.[213] NYHA-FC IIIb/IV pa-

TABLE 7.12 — β-BLOCKERS IN HEART FAILURE: MORTALITY END POINT TRIALS

Trial	Drugs	Control	Goal
BEST[31]	Bucindolol	Placebo	Mortality reduction: neutral NYHA-FC III-IV
CAPRICORN[50]	Carvedilol	Placebo	Mortality reduction: benefit post-MI
CIBIS-II[61,62,101,160]	Bisoprolol	Placebo	Mortality reduction: benefit NYHA-FC II-III
COMET[21,22,88,108,261]	Carvedilol	Metoprolol (short-acting dose)	Carvedilol was superior to short-acting, low-dose metoprolol
COPERNICUS[213]	Carvedilol	Placebo	Mortality reduction: benefit NYHA-FC IIIb-IV
MERIT-HF[129,191]	Metoprolol	Placebo	Mortality reduction: benefit NYHA-FC II-III

Abbreviations: BEST, β-Blocker Evaluation of Survival Trial; COMET, Carvedilol or Metoprolol European Trial; COPERNICUS, Carvedilol Prospective Randomized Cumulative Survival [trial]; MERIT-HF, Metoprolol CR/XL Randomized Intervention Trial in Heart Failure; MI, myocardial infarction; NYHA-FC, New York Heart Association functional class.

7

tients who had been adequately diuresed were begun on carvedilol with impressive results. In view of these data, clinicians should consider prescribing β-blockers, specifically carvedilol, for patients with advanced HF when well controlled from a volume perspective. The MERIT-HF study compared metoprolol with placebo in NYHA-FC II/III patients demonstrating substantive benefit with long-acting metoprolol.[129] The CIBIS-II trial[61,62,101,160] studied bisoprolol in a patient population similar to that in MERIT-HF and also demonstrated significant benefit. Finally, as alluded to earlier, COMET compared carvedilol with short-acting metoprolol.[21,22,88,108,238,261] This study showed that short-acting metoprolol is inferior to carvedilol.

Table 7.13 provides helpful hints for starting carvedilol or metoprolol. Patient selection for carvedilol and metoprolol should include those with mild-to-moderate CHF, and for carvedilol, stable severe HF patients who are not congested. Patients should be receiving an ACEI, usually a diuretic, and often digoxin. Starting β-blockers in patients hospitalized for decompensated CHF prior to discharge is safe and important when stabilization has occurred.

The starting dose of long-acting metoprolol is 12.5 mg daily and for carvedilol, 3.125 mg twice daily. This dose can be given either at bedtime or in the morning. If the first dose of these drugs is well tolerated, one should double the subsequent dose after 1 to 4 weeks of observation. Further dose doubling should occur until targets are reached, which are 25 mg twice daily for carvedilol and 200 mg daily for long-acting metoprolol. Symptomatic hypotension while taking carvedilol can sometimes be alleviated by instructing the patient to take this medication with meals. Another helpful tactic is to initially administer carvedilol 2 hours or so before or after other vasoactive agents. Patients rarely need to do this after steady-state drug doses have been achieved. When using long-acting metoprolol, we sometimes give the β-blocker in the morning and use a long-acting ACEI in the evening. As previously mentioned, if hypotension is particularly problematic, consider reducing diuretic or other vasodilator doses. Sometimes one has to down-titrate β-blockers but this should be done only when all else fails. Worsening symptoms of congestion (edema, weight gain, dyspnea syndromes) should be addressed by intensifying salt and fluid restriction, increasing diuretic doses, or perhaps by decreasing the β-blocker dose.

Significant bradycardia (heart rates consistently <60 or 65 beats per minute with associated symptoms) should be addressed by first making certain that concomitant medications are not contributing to the problem. One should monitor digoxin levels and decrease digoxin dose if necessary. Consider reducing amiodarone doses or eliminating the drug entirely. Verapamil or diltiazem should be stopped in HF patients. Finally, one may be forced to back-titrate the β-blocker dose. However, we would consider pacing prior to doing this, particularly if there is a wide QRS complex and a biventricular cardiac resynchronizing device can be used. Pacemaker implantation allows one to dose β-blockers more aggressively. Admittedly, this approach has not been extensively studied and some data suggest that simple AV sequential pacing can cause problems (see Chapter 10, *Arrhythmia and Electrophysiologic Considerations*).

Angiotensin II Receptor Blockers

Angiotensin II receptor blockers (**Table 7.14**) have been the focus of several recently completed clinical trials. As discussed in Chapter 5, *Clinical Trials Shaping Heart Failure Therapeutics*, today's knowledge base suggests that valsartan (Diovan) and candesartan (Atacand) have an important role in treating HF patients.

199

TABLE 7.13 — STARTING β-BLOCKERS* IN HEART FAILURE

- Patient selection:
  - Mild-to-moderate heart failure (HF)
  - Already receiving angiotensin-converting enzyme inhibitor (ACEI), usually a diuretic, often digoxin, and sometimes an aldosterone antagonist
  - Not recommended initially in patients hospitalized with decompensated HF or who have significant hypotension, pulmonary congestion, or problematic bradycardia (start drug after resolution of these difficulties even if patient is still hospitalized)
- Dosage:
  - Carvedilol:
    › Start with 3.125 mg bid with meals for 2 weeks or so
    › Counsel the patient about side effects after initial dose and after each dose increase (can have the patient take first dose or increased dose at bedtime)
    › If the first dose is tolerated well, increase to 6.25 mg bid after 1 to 4 weeks
    › Double the dose every 1 to 4 weeks until target reached (slower up-titration may be required); 25 mg bid in patients who weigh ≤85 kg or 50 mg bid in patients weighing >85 kg
    › Tell the patient to take carvedilol with meals
  - Long-acting metoprolol:
    › Start 12.5 or 25 mg (more stable patient) once daily (can take at bedtime)
    › Double dose regularly as above
    › Target dose is 200 mg qd
- Dealing with side effects during titration:
  - Vasodilating effects (dizziness or light-headedness)
    › Give carvedilol with food
    › Give β-blocker 2 hours before or after other vasoactive agents
    › Give ACEIs at bedtime and carvedilol bid or long-acting metoprolol in the morning (or reverse)

> › Consider reducing diuretic or other vasodilator doses temporarily
> › Reduce β-blocker dose only when other tactics fail
> › May require no attention, as symptoms often self-limiting
- Worsening HF (edema, weight gain, dyspnea):
  - Intensify salt restriction
  - Increase diuretic dose
  - Reduce β-blocker dose only when other tactics fail
- Significant bradycardia (consistently <60 to 65 beats/min with symptoms):
  - Monitor digoxin levels
  - Reduce digoxin dose
  - Reduce or eliminate amiodarone
  - Eliminate verapamil or diltiazem
  - Reduce β-blocker dose only when other tactics fail
  - Consider pacer (particularly biventricular unit if QRS >120 msec)

* Either carvedilol (Coreg) or long-acting metoprolol (Toprol-XL) is our drug of first choice, and we avoid low-dose, short-acting metoprolol.

The results of the recently completed CHARM trial programs indicate that candesartan significantly reduces mortality and morbidity in patients intolerant of ACEIs.[110] A similar observation was made in a subset of the V-HeFT Study.[68] The CHARM-Added trial also indicated that CHF patients remaining symptomatic despite aggressive baseline therapies, often including ACEIs, β-blockers, and aldosterone antagonists, improved with addition of the ARB candesartan to the protocol.[189]

The suggestion of an adverse interaction when ACEIs, β-blockers, and an ARB were combined noted in V-HeFT[68] was not found in CHARM. Although ARBs should not be considered equivalent to ACEIs in the treatment of CHF and should not be used as primary therapy in patients in whom an ACEI has not been tried, they may add value when used in the fash-

TABLE 7.14 — MEDICATIONS COMMONLY USED FOR HEART FAILURE: ANGIOTENSIN RECEPTOR BLOCKERS

Generic (Trade) Drug	Initial Dose (mg)	Target Dose (mg)	Maximum Dose (mg)	Major Adverse Reactions
Candesartan (Atacand)*	16 qd	32 qd	32 qd	Hypotension, hyperkalemia, rash, renal insufficiency
Losartan (Cozaar)	25 qd	100 qd	50 bid or 100 qd	
Valsartan (Diovan)*	80 qd	160 qd	320 qd	

* Agents with convincing data indicating benefit in certain heart failure populations.

ion delineated above. It may be the case that the beneficial effects of ARBs do not represent a simple "drug class effect." The two ARBs best studied in CHF populations with positive results are candesartan and valsartan.

Other Medications Used for Heart Failure

Table 7.15 lists other medications commonly used for HF, including digoxin (Lanoxin), HYD (Apresoline), and several long-acting oral nitrate compounds. Digoxin does reduce HF hospitalizations.[33,46,81,174,197,247,275] The drug appears to have an overall neutral effect on mortality. Important principles of prescribing digoxin are listed in **Table 7.16** and emphasize the fact that the lowest dose is likely the most reasonable dose (0.125 mg daily). We obtain digoxin levels only when toxicity is suspected (patients presenting with cryptogenic nausea, anorexia, confusion, visual disturbances, or arrhythmias). Serial digoxin levels are unnecessary. Hypokalemia and hypomagnesemia enhance digoxin toxicity while amiodarone and renal insufficiency increase digoxin levels and can also contribute to toxicity.

Table 7.17 summarizes medications other than ACEIs and β-blockers that are useful to treat hypertension or high-normal blood pressure in patients with HF.[36,79,154,164,243,265,272] This includes the calcium channel blocking agents amlodipine (Norvasc) and felodipine (Plendil). In general, we do not recommend calcium channel blocker therapy for patients with significant cardiac dysfunction. Amlodipine and felodipine remain possible exceptions: clinical trials have indicated that most patients with HF tolerate these agents without substantial deterioration.

The addition of HYD to an ACEI program will often result in symptomatic improvement and improved

TABLE 7.15 — OTHER MEDICATIONS COMMONLY USED FOR HEART FAILURE

Generic (Trade) Drug	Initial Dose (mg)	Target Dose (mg)	Maximum Dose (mg)	Major Adverse Reactions
Digoxin				
Digoxin, Lanoxin	0.125 qd	0.125-0.25 qd	0.25 qd	Cardiac arrhythmias, confusion, nausea, anorexia, visual disturbances
Hydralazine				
Apresoline	10-25 tid	75 tid	100 tid	Headache, nausea, dizziness, tachycardia, lupuslike syndrome
Long-Acting Oral Nitrates				
Isosorbide dinitrate (Isodril, Sorbitrate)	10 tid	40 tid	80 tid	Headache, hypotension, flushing
Isosorbide mononitrate (Ismo)	20 bid	20 bid	20 bid	

TABLE 7.16 — DIGOXIN THERAPY: ISSUES TO CONSIDER

- Start at lowest dose for everyone—0.125 mg
- Only obtain digoxin levels if toxicity suspected:
  - Cryptogenic nausea
  - Anorexia
  - Confusion
  - Visual disturbances
  - Arrhythmia
- Serial digoxin levels usually unnecessary
- Hypokalemia enhances toxicity
- Ensure adequate magnesium/potassium levels
- Remember that amiodarone and renal insufficiency enhance toxicity

blood pressure control. HYD may be given 3 times daily on an every-8-hour schedule. In practical terms, the most commonly encountered problem with HYD is difficulty maintaining the dosing schedule. However, chronic HYD administration can be associated with hypersensitivity reactions. Clonidine offers an attractive alternative when given via a transdermal patch since dosing is simplified. This central-acting α-adrenergic blocking agent, however, often causes sedation, dry mouth, and blurred vision. Some patients develop a contact dermatitis from the clonidine patch. Some investigators have suggested adding an ARB to baseline HF protocols (including protocols with ACEIs) to either treat *de novo* HF or assist with lowering the blood pressure. This strategy, as alluded to, has proven effective.

Anticoagulants

Anticoagulation is often necessary in patients with HF. These HF patients frequently have AF, which mandates warfarin prescription. Some practitioners believe routine anticoagulation is important simply be-

TABLE 7.17 — MEDICATIONS OTHER THAN ACE INHIBITORS AND β-BLOCKERS USED TO TREAT HYPERTENSION OR HIGH-NORMAL BLOOD PRESSURE IN PATIENTS WITH HEART FAILURE

Generic (Trade) Drug	Initial Dose (mg)	Maximum Dose (mg)	Major Adverse Reactions
Alpha₁-Adrenergic Blockers			
Doxazosin (Cardura)	1 qd	16 qd	Postural hypotension, dizziness, syncope, headache
Prazosin (Minipress)	1 tid	10 tid	
Terazosin (Hytrin)	1 qd	20 qd	
Angiotensin II Receptor Blockers			
Candesartan (Atacand)	16 qd	32 qd	Hypotension
Irbesartan (Avapro)	150 qd	300 qd	
Losartan (Cozaar)	25 qd	100 qd	Hypotension, mild renal insufficiency
Olmesartan (Benicar)	20 qd	40 qd	Hypotension
Telmisartan (Micardis)	40 qd	80 qd	
Valsartan (Diovan)	80 qd	320 qd	

Calcium Channel Blockers			
Amlodipine (Norvasc)	2.5 qd	10 qd	Hypotension, edema, headache
Felodipine (Plendil)	2.5 qd	10 qd	
Centrally-Acting Alpha Blockers			
Clonidine tablets (Catapres)	0.1 bid	0.6 bid	Sedation, dry mouth, blurry vision
Clonidine patch	0.1 weekly	0.3 weekly	*Same as clonidine*; contact dermatitis
Guanabenz (Wytensin)	4 bid	64 bid	Similar to clonidine
Guanfacine (Tenex)	1 qd	3 qd	
Direct Vasodilators			
Hydralazine (Apresoline)	10 tid	75 tid	Headache, nausea, dizziness, tachycardia, lupuslike syndrome
Minoxidil	2.5 qd	80 qd	Fluid retention, hair growth, thrombocytopenia, leukopenia

cause of a low EF. Individuals with mechanical heart valves should, of course, receive anticoagulation titrated to recommended standards. LVD alone is not a strong indication for chronic oral anticoagulation, but one might consider this tactic in individuals who have experienced thrombophlebitis, or prior embolic episodes or who have LV mural thrombi or left atrial clot identified. In patients with left atrial enlargement or with significant degrees of functional mitral regurgitation, ambulatory monitoring is indicated in order to document paroxysms of AF for which anticoagulation therapy is indicated.

As **Figure 7.7** indicates, multiple drug interactions occur with warfarin. Patients must be aware that response to warfarin will depend on multiple variables, including gastrointestinal absorption, hepatic perfusion, and congestion, and the many other drugs to which most of these individuals are exposed. Patients should be taught the importance of frequent international normalized ratio (INR) monitoring and should be encouraged to actively participate in their anticoagulant therapeutic decisions.

In summary, each of the major classes of drugs required for HF management has unique properties that require the treating physician to understand the pharmacology of the agents used, the circumstances in which therapy can be initiated, and the subtleties of titrating drugs to achieve target doses without untoward effects. Unfortunately, aggressive therapy with its concomitant benefits of morbidity and mortality reduction requires complicated polypharmacy protocols; this is addressed in Chapter 8, *Rational Polypharmacy*.

FIGURE 7.7 — HEART FAILURE MANAGEMENT: ORAL ANTICOAGULATION ALGORITHM

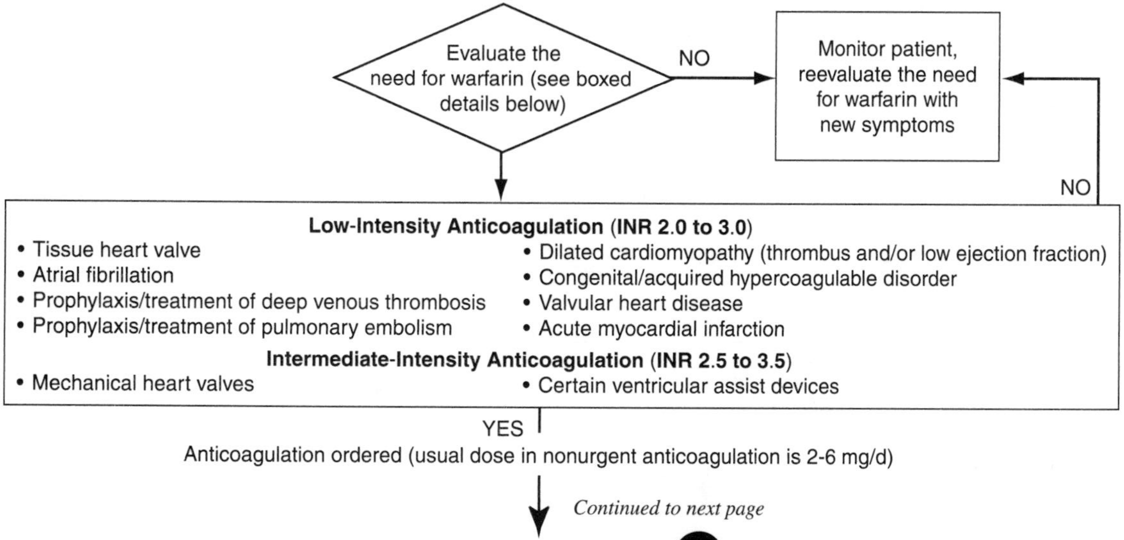

Evaluate the need for warfarin (see boxed details below)

NO → Monitor patient, reevaluate the need for warfarin with new symptoms

NO ↑

YES

Anticoagulation ordered (usual dose in nonurgent anticoagulation is 2-6 mg/d)

Continued to next page →

Low-Intensity Anticoagulation (INR 2.0 to 3.0)

- Tissue heart valve
- Atrial fibrillation
- Prophylaxis/treatment of deep venous thrombosis
- Prophylaxis/treatment of pulmonary embolism

- Dilated cardiomyopathy (thrombus and/or low ejection fraction)
- Congenital/acquired hypercoagulable disorder
- Valvular heart disease
- Acute myocardial infarction

Intermediate-Intensity Anticoagulation (INR 2.5 to 3.5)

- Mechanical heart valves
- Certain ventricular assist devices

NO

7

Continued from previous page

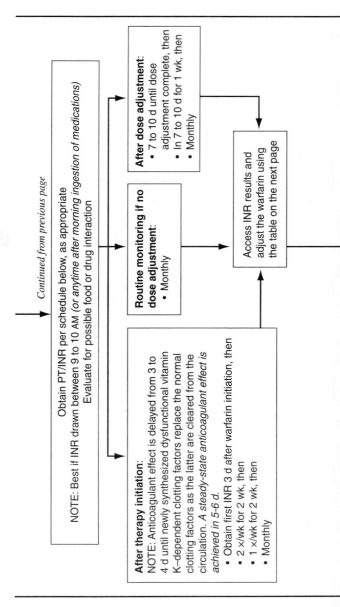

Obtain PT/INR per schedule below, as appropriate
NOTE: Best if INR drawn between 9 to 10 AM *(or anytime after morning ingestion of medications)*
Evaluate for possible food or drug interaction

After therapy initiation:
NOTE: Anticoagulant effect is delayed from 3 to 4 d until newly synthesized dysfunctional vitamin K–dependent clotting factors replace the normal clotting factors as the latter are cleared from the circulation. *A steady-state anticoagulant effect is achieved in 5-6 d.*
- Obtain first INR 3 d after warfarin initiation, then
- 2 x/wk for 2 wk, then
- 1 x/wk for 2 wk, then
- Monthly

Routine monitoring if no dose adjustment:
- Monthly

After dose adjustment:
- 7 to 10 d until dose adjustment complete, then
- In 7 to 10 d for 1 wk, then
- Monthly

Access INR results and adjust the warfarin using the table on the next page

Warfarin Dose Adjustment (mg) — Use column that reflects Desired Range		
INR	**2.0 to 3.0**	**2.5 to 3.5**
<1.5	↑ Weekly dose by 5% to 20%	↑ Weekly dose by 15% to 20%
1.5 to 2.0	↑ Weekly dose by 5% to 10%	↑ Weekly dose by 5% to 15%
2.0 to 2.5	Therapeutic; no change in dose	↑ Weekly dose by 5% to 10%
2.5 to 3.0	Therapeutic; no change in dose	Therapeutic; no change in dose
3.0 to 3.5	↓ Weekly dose by 5% to 10%	Therapeutic; no change in dose
3.5 to 4.0	Hold 1 dose. ↓ Weekly dose by 5% to 10%	↓ Weekly dose by 5% to 10%
4.0 to 6.0	Hold 1 to 2 doses. ↓ Weekly dose by 10% to 20%	Hold 1 to 2 doses. ↓ Weekly dose by 5% to 15%
>6 to <10	A) Assess for signs of bleeding, such as nosebleeds, bleeding from gums, unusual bleeding or bruising, red or dark brown urine, red or tar-black stools B) If vitamin K is ordered, the dose is: • 1-2 mg subcutaneously; check INR in 24 h • If INR remains high, give vitamin K 0.5 mg subcutaneously; repeat INR in 24 h and follow table above if INR is <6 • If INR remains >6 after 2 doses of vitamin K, consult with physician	
>10	A) Assess for signs of bleeding, such as nosebleeds, bleeding from gums, unusual bleeding or bruising, red or dark brown urine, red or tar-black stools B) Consult with physician. If vitamin K is ordered, the dose is: • 3 mg subcutaneously; check INR in 6 h • If INR remains >10, give vitamin K 3 mg subcutaneously; repeat INR in 6 to 24 h and follow table above if INR is <10, notify physician if INR remains ≥6 • If INR remains >10 after 2 doses of vitamin K, consider fresh-frozen plasma infusion	

Continued to next page

7

Continued from previous page

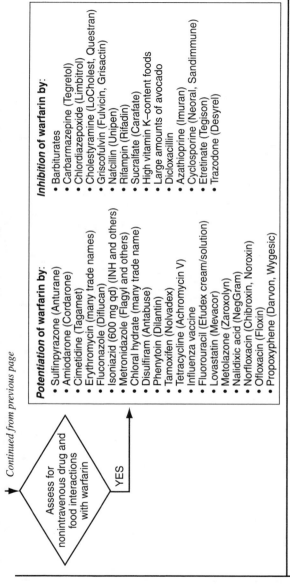

Assess for
nonintravenous drug and
food interactions
with warfarin

YES

Potentiation of warfarin by:
- Sulfinpyrazone (Anturane)
- Amiodarone (Cordarone)
- Cimetidine (Tagamet)
- Erythromycin (many trade names)
- Fluconazole (Diflucan)
- Isoniazid (600 mg qd) (INH and others)
- Metronidazole (Flagyl and others)
- Chloral hydrate (many trade name)
- Disulfiram (Antabuse)
- Phenytoin (Dilantin)
- Tamoxifen (Nolvadex)
- Tetracycline (Achromycin V)
- Influenza vaccine
- Fluorouracil (Efudex cream/solution)
- Lovastatin (Mevacor)
- Metolazone (Zaroxolyn)
- Nalidixic acid (NegGram)
- Norfloxacin (Chibroxin, Noroxin)
- Ofloxacin (Floxin)
- Propoxyphene (Darvon, Wygesic)

Inhibition of warfarin by:
- Barbiturates
- Carbamazepine (Tegretol)
- Chlordiazepoxide (Limbitrol)
- Cholestyramine (LoCholest, Questran)
- Griscofulvin (Fulvicin, Grisactin)
- Nafcillin (Unipen)
- Rifampin (Rifadin)
- Sucralfate (Carafate)
- High vitamin K-content foods
- Large amounts of avocado
- Dicloxacillin
- Azathioprine (Imuran)
- Cyclosporine (Neoral, Sandimmune)
- Etretinate (Tegison)
- Trazodone (Desyrel)

Abbreviations: INR, international normalized ratio; PT, prothrombin time.

212

8   Rational Polypharmacy

The rational management of heart failure (HF) patients, with its inevitable polypharmacy practices, requires integrating functional, imaging, clinical, and laboratory data to help titrate drug therapy, appropriately classify the patient according to the American College of Cardiology/American Heart Association (ACC/AHA) and the New York Heart Association functional class (NYHA-FC), and make decisions about surgical and device management. The introduction of B-type natriuretic peptide (BNP) assays offers clinicians a new tool with which to guide HF management.[176] Two small trials of BNP-guided therapy for HF are summarized in **Table 8**.1. Both have shown encouraging results. In addition, data from V-HeFT, which included 4300 patients, underscore that changes in BNP (and plasma norepinephrine) are associated with changes in mortality and morbidity. The investigators emphasize the importance of these levels as surrogate markers in HF.[13]

Inevitably, management of patients with HF will require multiple drugs. **Figure 8**.1 presents results from the pooled analysis of the PROVED[297,317] and RADIANCE[215,317] trials. These trials showed that the likelihood of worsening symptomatic congestive heart failure (CHF) was lower in patients receiving triple-drug therapy with digoxin, an angiotensin-converting enzyme inhibitor (ACEI), and a diuretic than in any of the other groups. Particularly important was the observation that an ACEI and diuretic alone are inferior to the combination of the three drugs. In the SOLVD registry, HF patients received a median of four different drugs for HF, as well as additional medications for comorbidities such as diabetes, degenerative joint dis-

TABLE 8.1 — B-TYPE NATRIURETIC PEPTIDE–GUIDED HEART FAILURE THERAPY			
Authors	No. of Subjects	Duration (months)	Outcome
Murdoch et al	20	2	Significantly lower BNP levels with guided therapy
Troughton et al	69	9.5 (median)	Fewer deaths, admissions, and decompensation with guided therapy (27% vs 53%, $P = 0.034$)

Abbreviation: BNP, B-type natriuretic peptide.

Murdoch DR, et al. *Am Heart J.* 1999;138:1005-1006 and Troughton RW, et al. *Lancet.* 2000;355:1112-1113.

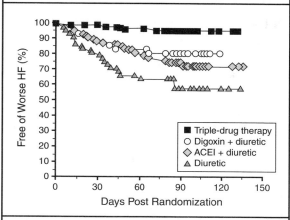

FIGURE 8.1 — LIKELIHOOD OF DETERIORATION IN HEART FAILURE

Legend:
- ■ Triple-drug therapy
- ○ Digoxin + diuretic
- ◇ ACEI + diuretic
- ▲ Diuretic

Abbreviations: ACEI, angiotensin-converting enzyme inhibitor; HF, heart failure.

Triple-drug therapy appears best in congestive heart failure (HF) patients. This sets the baseline foundation to which other HF drugs are added.

Modified from: Young JB, et al. *J Am Coll Cardiol*. 1998;32: 686-692.

8

ease, dyspepsia, or dysphoric syndromes. **Figure 8**.**2** demonstrates differences in medication use in the SOLVD registry (1990) and the SPICE registry (1997).[28,109,259] More patients, for example, were on ACEIs and β-blockers in the more contemporary SPICE registry, while fewer patients were taking calcium channel blockers and antiarrhythmic drugs.

Earlier diagnosis of asymptomatic or minimally symptomatic systolic left ventricular dysfunction (LVD) can be important. Earlier diagnosis will require fewer drugs. Diuretics, for example, are only indicated when congestion is present. In the patient with isolated systolic LVD, an ACEI in combination with a β-

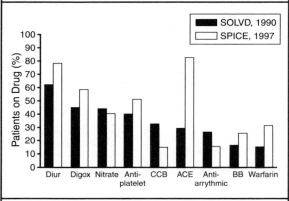

**FIGURE 8.2 — MEDICATION USE IN
SOLVD (1990) AND SPICE (1997) REGISTRIES**

Abbreviations: ACE, angiotensin-converting enzyme; BB, β-blocker; CCB, calcium channel blocker; Digox, digoxin; Diur, diuretic; SOLVD, Studies of Left Ventricular Dysfunction; SPICE, Study of Patients Intolerant of Converting Enzyme Inhibitors.

Drug-use patterns in two large registries of heart failure patients, demonstrating the large number of drugs used in these patients and the changing proportion of patients on ACE inhibitors, β-blockers, antiarrhythmic agents, and calcium channel blockers.

Bart BA, et al. *Eur Heart J.* 1999;20:1182-1190.

blocker would be indicated. Given the results of clinical trials, it is reasonable to speculate that therapy with ACEIs and β-blockers in these patients might prevent deterioration to a point of congestion that would mandate more complex polypharmacy.

We urge only starting or continuing drugs known to alleviate symptoms or reduce morbidity and mortality. As emphasized in Chapter 6, *General Treatment Approaches*, clinicians must avoid or discontinue drugs known to produce adverse events, such as antiarrhythmic agents, nonsteroidal anti-inflammatory drugs (NSAIDs), and insulin-sensitizing agents of the thiazolidinedione class (rosiglitazone/pioglitazone), when congestion is a problem. One should also avoid or stop drugs that are known to be neutral in their effects with respect to symptom reduction, morbidity, or mortality, and carefully match appropriate patients to treatments as dictated by clinical trial experience. Adding drugs or nutritional supplements to an already complicated polypharmacy regimen will only make therapeutic compliance more challenging.

Future pharmacogenomic approaches to the dilemma of polypharmacy will increase our ability to determine characteristics of individual patients that predict beneficial responses to the different drugs available for treating HF. Knowledge from such studies might perhaps eliminate the need for complicated polypharmacotherapeutic protocols.

Table 8.2 reinforces the concept of selecting drugs with beneficial actions. The ACC/AHA classification scheme underscores this strategy. β-Blockade reduces BNP levels in chronic HF, as does effective afterload reduction. In patients with systolic LVD who have echocardiographic evidence of moderate-to-severe mitral regurgitation, our strategy has been to titrate ACEI or ARB doses to target levels with modest background doses of β-blockers, then to slowly increase β-blocker doses if BNP levels remain elevated. In contrast, if mitral regurgitation is minimal or absent, we would reverse the order and initially titrate β-blockers to goal, then increase the background ACEI or ARB therapy as indicated by BNP levels. In either setting, diuretics should be used sparingly for overt congestion, not as a daily maintenance HF therapy. ACEIs, β-blockers, and probably aldosterone antagonists are important to prevent or modify disease progression and, specifically, cardiac remodeling.

TABLE 8.2 — RATIONAL POLYPHARMACY CONSIDERATIONS

Preventing/Modifying Disease Progression
- Angiotensin-converting enzyme inhibitors
- Angiotensin receptor blockers
- β-Blockers
- Aldosterone antagonists

Treatment of Concomitant Processes/Comorbidities
- Coronary artery disease:
  - Antiplatelet agents (ASA/clopidogrel)
  - Statins
- Hypertension:
  - Vasodilators
  - Thiazide diuretics
- Diabetes mellitus:
  - Insulin rather than thiazolidinediones in congested patients
- Gout:
  - Allopurinol (*not* NSAIDs)
- Atrial fibrillation:
  - Anticoagulation
  - Rate control
  - Rhythm control
- Chronic obstructive pulmonary disease:
  - Positive airway pressure devices
  - Bronchodilators
  - Antibiotics
  - Influenza/pneumonia shots
- Sleep apnea:
  - Continuous positive airway pressure devices

Treatment of Symptoms
- Digoxin (low dose)
- Nocturnal nitrates (long-acting)
- Diuretics (intermittent, weight-adjusted doses)

Abbreviations: ASA, acetylsalicylic acid; NSAID, non-steroid anti-inflammatory drug.

Treatment of comorbidities that contribute to disease progression must include addressing coronary artery disease with antiplatelet agents (eg, aspirin or clopidogrel) and statins in addition to effective β blockade. Patients who have objective evidence of myocardial ischemia and substantial viability should be considered for revascularization, if possible. Treating hypertension dramatically attenuates morbidity and mortality when LV dysfunction is present. When managing a patient with diabetes mellitus, one should consider insulin therapy rather than drugs that might predispose to fluid retention. In patients with atrial fibrillation, anticoagulation and rate and rhythm control are important. Some patients with chronic obstructive pulmonary disease, reactive airway disease, or sleep apnea syndromes respond nicely to therapies aimed at improving gas exchange and respiratory function. This generally helps to attenuate HF.

BNP-guided management might help minimize many familiar problems associated with overdiuresis with each patient's values used as his/her own controls. The ability to check BNP levels and to estimate right ventricular systolic pressure from the echocardiogram will provide objective data about the adequacy of diuretic doses in controlling filling pressures. **Table 8.3** summarizes some practical approaches to HF medication protocols when patients are taking several agents and complications such as orthostatic hypotension are noted. We deal with orthostatic hypotension using a three-step approach. First, be sure the problem is significant and not just a tolerable nuisance. Reassurance and counseling about flexing the calves immediately on standing and about not standing immobile for sustained periods helps. Reminders about the impact of good medical therapy on the prognosis of HF eliminate most complaints. Support hosiery may also help. Reduction in diuretic therapy should be the first pharmacologic maneuver if the patient is not congested

TABLE 8.3 — A PRACTICAL HEART FAILURE MEDICATION PROTOCOL

Breakfast (8 AM)	Dinner (7 PM)	Bedtime
ACEI	(? bid agent)	—
β-Blocker	—	β-Blocker
Loop diuretic	(? Extra)	—
Digoxin	—	—
—	—	Statin
(? Extra)	—	Long-acting nitrate
—	Aspirin	—
Other agents	Other agents	Other agents

Abbreviation: ACEI, angiotensin-converting enzyme inhibitor.

and, particularly, if the BNP is low or normal. Rarely, changes in the drug-administration program separating vasoactive drugs times may help. We sometimes use a long-acting β-blocker in the morning and a long-acting ACEI in the evening or vice versa. Of course, the downside of spacing medications throughout the day is that patients are confronted with complex protocols that could negatively impact compliance.

Figure 8.3 presents a hypotension treatment algorithm. Because many of the drugs used reduce afterload and blood pressure, dizziness, or wobbling when standing can be problematic. Patients with relatively low blood pressure frequently complain of malaise and fatigue. Often, when orthostatic symptoms are noted, severe fatigue can also be present, and this can cause the need to sit and rest when exercising. Supine systolic blood pressure consistently <80 mm Hg should also prompt evaluation of postural hypotension. Postural hypotension is present if the standing systolic blood pressure decreases from the supine systolic blood pressure by ≥15 mm Hg and/or the heart rate increases by >10 beats/min (this response can be attenuated by β-blockers). Note whether standing precipitates symptoms. If the patient is not volume overloaded, the first step is to decrease diuretics. When volume overload is present in a setting of orthostatic hypotension, patients usually require hospitalization for optimization of therapeutic protocols. Every effort must be made to avoid decreasing doses of ACEIs and β-blockers.

Figure 8.4 presents an algorithm to help with managing renal dysfunction in the setting of polypharmacy. Renal dysfunction can be challenging, but like hypotension, it must be reviewed in the context of the patient's volume status and concomitant medications. One should search for reversible causes of azotemia, such as over-the-counter NSAID ingestion, antibiotics, volume depletion, urinary tract infections, and obstructive uropathy. Only when other problems have been excluded should ACEIs and vasodilators be decreased.

In summary, polypharmacy is required to successfully manage HF. The simplest possible management program is most likely to succeed. The clinician must be willing to take some extra time to understand the patient's daily routine. Part of the art of successful HF therapy includes giving clear, unequivocal instructions about how and when to take medications. We emphasize taking diuretics, when needed, early in the morning and returning to bed for an hour or two to get the benefits of enhanced renal perfusion from supine posture. Even with long-acting drugs, we try to space them at 12-hour intervals to maintain stable drug levels and to make the morning and evening doses similar. Nonpharmacologic therapy with diet, lifestyle modifications, and exercise substantially decreases the complexity of drug management.

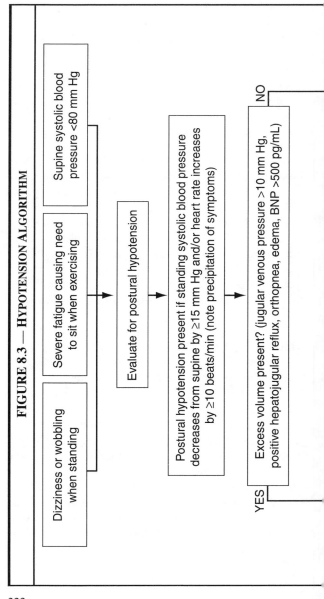

FIGURE 8.3 — HYPOTENSION ALGORITHM

Dizziness or wobbling when standing

Severe fatigue causing need to sit when exercising

Supine systolic blood pressure <80 mm Hg

Evaluate for postural hypotension

Postural hypotension present if standing systolic blood pressure decreases from supine by ≥15 mm Hg and/or heart rate increases by ≥10 beats/min (note precipitation of symptoms)

Excess volume present? (jugular venous pressure >10 mm Hg, positive hepatojugular reflux, orthopnea, edema, BNP >500 pg/mL)

YES   NO

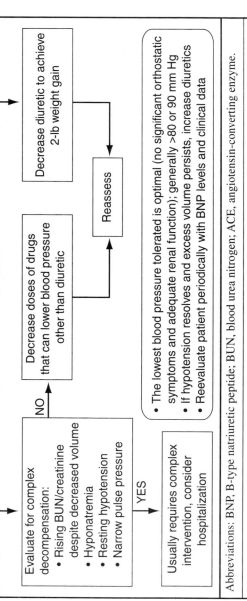

Evaluate for complex decompensation:
- Rising BUN/creatinine despite decreased volume
- Hyponatremia
- Resting hypotension
- Narrow pulse pressure

NO → Decrease doses of drugs that can lower blood pressure other than diuretic

YES

Usually requires complex intervention, consider hospitalization

Reassess

Decrease diuretic to achieve 2-lb weight gain

- The lowest blood pressure tolerated is optimal (no significant orthostatic symptoms and adequate renal function); generally >80 or 90 mm Hg
- If hypotension resolves and excess volume persists, increase diuretics
- Reevaluate patient periodically with BNP levels and clinical data

Abbreviations: BNP, B-type natriuretic peptide; BUN, blood urea nitrogen; ACE, angiotensin-converting enzyme.

When approaching patients with hypotension, one must assess the degree of excessive vasodilation vs volume overload. Every effort must be made to avoid decreasing doses of ACE inhibitors and β-blockers if at all possible.

8

223

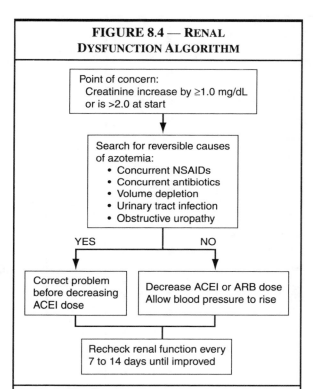

FIGURE 8.4 — RENAL DYSFUNCTION ALGORITHM

Point of concern:
Creatinine increase by ≥1.0 mg/dL or is >2.0 at start

Search for reversible causes of azotemia:
- Concurrent NSAIDs
- Concurrent antibiotics
- Volume depletion
- Urinary tract infection
- Obstructive uropathy

YES → Correct problem before decreasing ACEI dose

NO → Decrease ACEI or ARB dose Allow blood pressure to rise

Recheck renal function every 7 to 14 days until improved

Abbreviations: ACEI, angiotensin-converting enzyme inhibitor; ARB, angiotension receptor blocker; NSAID, nonsteroidal anti-inflammatory drug.

Renal dysfunction can be challenging to manage in the heart failure setting, but like hypotension, it must be reviewed in the context of a patient's status and concomitant medications that might produce azotemia.

Treatment of Decompensated or Refractory Heart Failure

Introduction

We define "decompensated" heart failure (HF) as an abrupt sustained increase or worsening of at least one New York Heart Association functional class (NYHA-FC) with objective evidence of intravascular volume overload or elevated left ventricular (LV) filling pressure. **Table 9**.1 lists various features of decompensated HF.

Physical examination of a decompensated patient often demonstrates:

- Resting tachycardia
- Resting tachypnea
- Vasoconstriction (cold hands and feet).

Signs of volume overload include:

- Jugular venous distention
- Hepatojugular reflux
- Peripheral edema
- Pulmonary rales
- Pleural effusions
- Ascites.

Substantial pulmonary congestion may be present *without* rales or jugular venous distention. Tricuspid insufficiency makes jugular vein infections challenging. A pulsatile liver is sometimes noted and hepatic tenderness often is present. Impaired mental acuity, apnea with periodic respirations, anxiety, apprehension, and depression are also significant findings in HF de-

TABLE 9.1 — FEATURES OF DECOMPENSATED CONGESTIVE HEART FAILURE

Physical
- Resting tachycardia
- Hypotension (sometimes hypertension):
  - Vasoconstriction (cold hands/feet) with hypotension
- Signs of volume overload:
  - Jugular venous distention
  - Hepatojugular reflux
  - Peripheral leg edema
- Rales (may *not* be present)
- Pulsatile liver
- Hepatic tenderness
- Impaired mental acuity
- Apnea/periodic respirations
- Anxiety/apprehension, depression

Hemodynamics
- Low cardiac index
- Low mixed venous oxygen saturation
- Elevated pulmonary capillary wedge pressures (>20 mm Hg)
- Large V wave if in normal sinus rhythm
- Large regurgitant wave with mitral regurgitation
- Altered thoracic impedance square-wave response to Valsalva's maneuver
- Narrow pulse pressure

Laboratory Findings
- Significant elevation of circulating B-type natriuretic peptide (BNP) levels
- Radiographic signs of pulmonary venous hypertension (may be absent)
- Prerenal azotemia
- Hyponatremia
- Hyperkalemia
- Acidosis
- Sometimes alkalosis
- Ventricular or atrial arrhythmias

compensation. Hemodynamics include a low cardiac index and low mixed venous oxygen (O_2) saturation, with elevated pulmonary capillary wedge pressure. Altered thoracic impedance and a "square-wave" response to Valsalva's maneuver are common manifestations of high left heart filling pressures. Narrow pulse pressure is a particularly dire sign.

Laboratory findings associated with severe decompensated HF often include:

- Elevated B-type natriuretic peptide (BNP) levels (>800 pg/mL)
- Radiographic signs of pulmonary venous hypertension (this may be absent despite significant wedge and pulmonary artery pressure elevation)
- Prerenal azotemia
- Hyponatremia
- Hypokalemia
- Acidosis (sometimes alkalosis)
- Ventricular or atrial arrhythmias.

The Acute Decompensated Heart Failure National Registry (ADHERE) database is a national observational registry of patients hospitalized with acute decompensated HF. An interim analysis from this database presented at the 7th Annual Scientific Meeting of the Heart Failure Society of America[97] found that blood urea nitrogen (BUN) >43 mg/dL is the best single predictor for hospital mortality.

The recent Food and Drug Administration (FDA) approval of measurement of BNP levels as an aid to the diagnosis of HF has had an important impact on improving care for HF patients. **Figure 9.1** summarizes the pathophysiology of BNP elevations in HF. The "Breathing Not Properly" Multinational Study included 1586 subjects presenting to emergency departments complaining of dyspnea, and it confirmed that BNP levels >100 pg/mL are helpful in establishing a

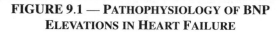

FIGURE 9.1 — PATHOPHYSIOLOGY OF BNP ELEVATIONS IN HEART FAILURE

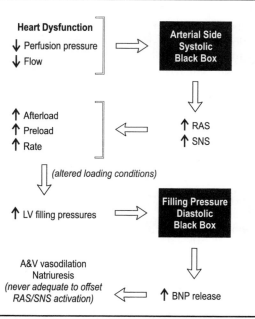

Abbreviation: A, arterial; BNP, B-type natriuretic peptide; RAS, renin-angiotensin system; SNS, sympathetic nervous system; V, venous.

diagnosis of HF, particularly when the clinical diagnosis is in question.[186]

In another report from the ADHERE registry,[310] 49% of the 16,074 patients who had LV function studies had an ejection fraction ≥0.40. BNP levels on admission averaged 647 pg/mL in the patients with preserved systolic function and 918 pg/mL in those with impaired systolic function ($n = 3628$ and 3436, respectively). The ADHERE registry data confirm that BNP determinations are useful in the diagnosis of HF with preserved systolic function.

Although physical examination and radiologic findings often suggest elevated LV filling pressure, substantial elevation of BNP levels provides additional objective data to support the diagnosis of HF. We strongly support the use of BNP levels in the evaluation, management, and prognostication of patients with dyspnea and suspected HF.

Predisposing Factors and Patterns for Decompensation

Table 9.2 lists factors predisposing to HF decompensation. It is important to consider concomitant cardiac problems, in particular, worsening ischemia, new myocardial infarction (MI), and new onset of atrial fibrillation. Uncontrolled hypertension and acute pulmonary embolism, as well as exacerbations of chronic obstructive pulmonary disease, can precipitate significant cardiac decompensation. Other issues to consider include inadequate medication protocols and use of medications (prescription, over-the-counter, or herbal) that predispose patients to fluid retention. Exposure to environmental temperature extremes and travel to altitude can also precipitate HF decompensation. Of course, noncompliance with treatment recommendations (diet, drugs, and physical activity) often precipitates problems.

Table 9.3 compares two patterns of HF decompensation with stable chronic findings. The sudden onset of pulmonary edema is generally seen with ischemia or hypertensive crisis; volume shifts, rather than volume overload, occur when sudden pulmonary artery pressure rises lead to pulmonary edema.

Hospital vs Home Care

Sometimes making the decision to admit a patient to the hospital for treatment of decompensated HF is

229

TABLE 9.2 — FACTORS PREDISPOSING TO HEART FAILURE DECOMPENSATION

Concomitant Disease States/Comorbidities
- Worsening ischemia or new infarction
- Hypertension not controlled
- Acute pulmonary embolism
- COPD decompensation
- Infection (bronchitis, pneumonia, cellulitis)
- Diabetic hyperglycemia/acidosis
- Hyperosmolar nonketotic state
- Electrolyte abnormalities (hyponatremia in particular)
- Renal insufficiency
- Anemia
- Hyper-/hypothyroidism (particularly with amiodarone)
- Obesity/hypoventilation (sleep apnea)
- Obesity/deconditioning
- Arrhythmias (particularly new atrial fibrillation)
- Acute valvular catastrophe (sudden severe mitral or aortic regurgitation)
- Malignancy with myocardial/pericardial metastases

Inadequate Medication Protocol
- Not enough diuretic
- Not using diuretic combinations
- Not at target ACEI, ARB, β-blocker dose

Use of Certain Medications
- Nonsteroidal anti-inflammatory agents
- Thiazolidinediones (rosiglitazone/pioglitazone)
- Certain chemotherapy agents

Exposure to Environmental Temperature Extremes

Travel to a Higher Altitude

Noncompliance With Treatment
- Diet
- Drugs
- Activity

Abbreviations: ACEI, angiotensin-converting enzyme inhibitor; ARB, angiotensin receptor blocker; COPD, chronic obstructive pulmonary disease.

difficult (**Table 9**.4). Findings that favor hospitalization include the acute onset of symptoms, a systolic blood pressure <90 mm Hg, heart rate consistently >100 beats/min, severe peripheral edema or hepatic congestion, medical noncompliance, and poor psychosocial support structures. Hyponatremia, hypokalemia, and azotemia also favor hospitalization, as do tachypnea, periodic respirations, and a narrow pulse pressure.

Home care requires strict adherence to a low-salt diet and fluid restriction (**Table 9**.5). Bed rest for at least 2 hours after oral diuretic administration and after the midday meal may help to mobilize fluid. Using twice-daily diuretics or combinations of diuretics (ie, premedication with metolazone at least an hour before furosemide) can help. Sometimes arranging home health care is advantageous if visiting nurses can give parenteral loop diuretics. Monitoring patients in the home environment does require careful attention and either frequent visits to the outpatient clinic or supervision by home health care teams.

Table 9.6 summarizes the therapeutic goals and interventions in hospitalized patients with acute decompensated HF. As data from new clinical trials, including the VMAC trial,[244] PRECEDENT trial,[42] and OPTIME-CHF study,[77] have indicated, parenteral vasodilator therapy for acute decompensated HF effectively decreases filling pressures and increases forward cardiac output in most patients. Clinically, it is critical to understand that vasodilator therapy alters loading conditions, *not* cardiac function. Vasodilator therapy, therefore, will not stabilize patients with end-stage HF and ventricular dysfunction at a stage where the heart cannot support the circulation even under optimal loading conditions. If these patients require temporary pharmacologic support, one must turn to positive inotropes (ie, dopamine or dobutamine) or "inodilators" (ie, milrinone). Inotrope prescription is unfortunately associated with problems, such as

TABLE 9.3 — COMPARISON OF ACUTE VS CHRONIC HEART FAILURE

Feature	Heart Failure		
	Acute	Decompensated Chronic	Stable Chronic
Symptom severity	Marked	Marked	Mild to moderate
Symptom onset	Sudden	Semiacute	Chronic
Pulmonary edema	Frequent	Frequent	Rare
Weight gain	None to mild	Marked	Frequent
Total body volume	No change or mild increase	Markedly increased	Increased
Cardiomegaly	Uncommon	Usual	Common
LV systolic function	Hypo-, normo-, or hypercontractile	Reduced	Markedly reduced
Wall stress	Elevated	Markedly elevated	Elevated
Activation of sympathetic nervous system	Marked	Marked	Mild to marked

Activation of RAAS	Acutely abnormal	Marked	Mild to marked
BNP levels	Generally 200-600 pg/mL; (in some patients may be **normal**)	Markedly elevated; >600 pg/mL (>1000 pg/mL in severely ill)	Compensated; usually 200-500 pg/mL
Acute ischemia	Common	Occasional	Rare
Hypertensive crisis	Common	Occasional	Rare
Reparable, remedial causative lesions	Common	Occasional	Occasional

Abbreviations: BNP, B-type natriuretic peptide; LV, left ventricular; RAAS, renin-angiotensin-aldosterone system.

9

TABLE 9.4 — HOSPITAL VS HOME CARE FOR DECOMPENSATED HEART FAILURE

Favors Hospitalization	Favors Home
NYHA-FC IV	NYHA-FC III
SBP <90 mm Hg	SBP >100 mm Hg
HR >100 bpm	HR <100 bpm
BNP levels >600 pg/mL	BNP levels <600 pg/mL
Edema ≥3+ or hepatic congestion	Edema ≤2+
Medically noncompliant and/or poor psychosocial support	Compliant patient with supportive psychosocial milieu
Tachypnea (RR >15-20)	Comfortable at rest (RR <15)
Periodic respirations	Normal breathing pattern
Narrow pulse pressure (proportion of pulse pressure <0.25)	Proportional pulse pressure >0.25
Hyponatremia	Normal sodium
Hyperkalemia	Normal potassium
Azotemia	Normal renal function

Abbreviations: BNP, B-type natriuretic peptide; HR, heart rate; NYHA-FC, New York Heart Association functional class; RR, relative risk; SBP, systolic blood pressure.

arrhythmias. In the vast majority of patients who experience acute decompensation, vasodilator therapy will fortunately result in rapid hemodynamic and symptomatic improvement.

Vasodilator therapy with either nesiritide or nitroprusside produces prompt decreases in neurohormonal activation. In contrast, diuretic monotherapy decreases filling pressures at the expense of forward cardiac output and glomerular filtration rate. The fall in intravascular volume and decrement in cardiac output

TABLE 9.5 — HOME CARE BASICS

Diet
- Strict salt, water limits

Activity
- Bed rest at least 2 h after po diuretics and after mid-day meal

*Drugs**
- Diuretics/combination diuretics bid (ie, premedication with metolazone 30 to 60 min before furosemide); consider parenteral tactics. **Decrease diuretics when stabilized!**

Monitoring
- Office and lab every 48 to 72 h

* In addition to other agents.

TABLE 9.6 — ACUTE HEART FAILURE: THERAPEUTIC GOALS AND INTERVENTIONS IN HOSPITALIZED PATIENTS

Treatment Goals	Pharmacologic Intervention
Reduce impedence to ventricular ejection and reduce wall stress	• Arteriolar/venous vasodilators • PDE inhibitors ("inodilators")
Reduce ventricular filling pressure	• Venous vasodilators • Diuretics • PDE inhibitors ("inodilators")
Increase contractility	• PDE inhibitors ("inodilators") • Sympathomimetics
Increase lusitropy	• Nesiritide • PDE inhibitors ("inodilators")
Increase coronary perfusion	• Nesiritide • Coronary vasodilators • PDE inhibitors ("inodilators")
Abbreviation: PDE, phosphodiesterase.	

9

associated with aggressive diuresis lead to further increases in renin-angiotensin system (RAS) activation, an undesirable outcome. Excessive diuresis in the HF patient then leads to inability to tolerate afterload reduction or angiotensin-converting enzyme (ACE) inhibition due to hypotension or worsening azotemia. Currently available clinical trials data support the early institution of effective vasodilator therapy supplemented by modest doses of diuretics in order to rapidly stabilize most acutely decompensated patients.[141,266,267]

Usually when a patient is admitted to the hospital for therapy, electrocardiographic monitoring (telemetry) is instituted to watch for potentially life-threatening arrhythmia (**Table 9.7**). Daily weight and fluid intake/output measured every nursing shift help determine net fluid balance. Supplemental oxygen (O_2) may help improve tissue oxygenation and lower pulmonary artery pressure if sleep apnea or periodic respirations are present. Salt and water restriction is crucial. Excessive volume and solute intake driven by increased thirst in HF will lead to hyponatremia and worsening congestive states. Giving medications every 8 or 12 hours will avoid reactivation or escape of neurohormonal blockade. Subcutaneous low molecular weight heparin administration may limit development of venous thrombosis. Ambulation, when possible, can also decrease thromboembolism risk.

Invasive Hemodynamic Monitoring

Although no guidelines exist for recommending invasive hemodynamic monitoring in patients with decompensated HF, we consider right-heart catheterization when there is a clinical picture of intravascular volume depletion with HF symptoms and particularly when hypotension and oliguria occur (**Table 9.8**).

TABLE 9.7 — STANDARD INTERVENTIONS IN HOSPITALIZED HEART FAILURE PATIENTS

Recommendation	Rationale
Telemetry	Potential for life-threatening arrhythmia
Daily weight/fluid intake and output measured every shift	Monitor net fluid balance
Supplemental oxygen	Improve tissue oxygenation
Salt and water restriction	Thirst often leads to continued water intake with hyponatremia
Every 8- or 12-h medications	Avoid reactivation or escape of neurohumoral blockade
Thromboembolic prophylaxis with subcutaneous low molecular weight heparin	Heart failure and limited activity predispose to venous thrombosis
Ambulation when possible/practical	Decrease thromboembolism risk

9

Right-heart catheterization is also helpful in evaluating the response to specific interventions and to optimize hemodynamics. This is generally accomplished by vasodilator infusion, although some patients may require inotrope support. In patients with cardiogenic shock, intra-aortic balloon counterpulsation support may be necessary, and in individuals who are candidates for cardiac transplantation, quickly moving to a ventricular assist device can be lifesaving. These decisions are facilitated by hemodynamic data.

Table 9.9 summarizes the benefits and potential problems of hemodynamic-guided parenteral drug therapy for decompensated HF.[76] The potential ben-

TABLE 9.8 — INDICATIONS FOR HEMODYNAMIC MONITORING IN HEART FAILURE

Consider Right-Heart Catheterization
- Evaluate hemodynamics—clinical picture of intravascular volume depletion with heart failure symptoms:
  - Hypotension
  - Oliguria
- Evaluate response to specific intervention (tailored therapeutics):
  - Inotrope and/or vasodilator infusion
  - Intra-aortic balloon pump support
- Physiologic monitoring (decreasing risk of adverse events during intervention):
  - Ventilatory support
  - Surgical procedure

efits include clarification of specific hemodynamic measures, allowing a more rapid tailoring of treatments, achieving better hemodynamic parameters, and allowing easier and safer up-titration of oral neurohormonal blocking agents with perhaps a shortening of hospital stay. Potential problems include complications of catheter insertion, complications of the catheter per se, potential for flawed data or data misinterpretation, and requirement for an intensive care unit (ICU), which is a more costly environment.

Common hemodynamic patterns noted in decompensated states are listed in **Table 9.10**. By knowing these findings, one can tailor therapy to improve any specific clinical situation. **Table 9.11** outlines hemodynamic effects of parenteral support agents commonly used in decompensated congestive HF.

Table 9.12 summarizes the side effects of parenterally administered inotropic and vasodilating agents.

TABLE 9.9 — ISSUES TO CONSIDER REGARDING HEMODYNAMIC-GUIDED CONTINUOUS-INFUSION PARENTERAL DRUG THERAPY FOR DECOMPENSATED CONGESTIVE HEART FAILURE

Potential Benefits	Potential Problems
Clarification of specific hemodynamic measures	Complications of catheter insertion
Allows faster tailoring of treatments	Complication of indwelling catheter
Helps in achieving optimal hemodynamic parameters	Potential for flawed data or data misinterpretation
Easier/safer to up-titrate oral neurohormonal blocking agents	Requires intensive care unit
Shortens hospital stay	Could be more costly

New Agents for Decompensated Heart Failure

Nesiritide is the first new parenteral agent approved by the FDA for HF treatment in over a decade and a half. It is a 32 amino acid peptide structurally identical to endogenous human BNP. Nesiritide binds to receptors on vascular smooth muscle and endothelial cells, producing balanced vasodilation through a guanosine monophosphate mechanism. Clearance also occurs at the vascular endothelial sites with a half-life of 18 to 20 minutes and is not dependent on renal or hepatic function.

In HF, the balanced vasodilator effects of nesiritide reduce pulmonary capillary wedge, pulmonary artery, and right atrial pressures and systemic vascular resistance. Redistribution of functional mitral regurgitant flow and improved loading conditions re-

TABLE 9.10 — COMMON HEMODYNAMIC PATTERNS IN DECOMPENSATED HEART FAILURE STATES

Heart Failure State	CO	PAP	PCWP	RAP	SVO_2	SVR
Acute pulmonary edema	Variable	Variable	Variable	→	Variable	Variable
Cardiogenic shock	→	↑→	↑→	←	↑↑	↑↑
Decompensated heart failure	→	↑↑	↑↑	←	←	←
Acute right ventricular failure	→	→↑	→↑	↑↑	←	←
Massive pulmonary embolism	→	←	↑	←	→	←
Acute aortic/mitral valve insufficiency	→	←	↑↑	→	→	←
Tamponade	→	←	←	←	→	←
Hypovolemic shock	→	→	→	→	→	←

Abbreviations: CO, cardiac ouput; PAP, pulmonary artery pressure; PCWP, pulmonary capillary wedge pressure; RAP, right atrial pressure; SVO_2, venous oxygen saturation; SVR, systemic vascular resistance.

sult in increased forward cardiac output. Nesiritide alone has modest natriuretic and diuretic effects, but it markedly enhances the response to loop diuretics. **Table 9.13** summarizes the hemodynamic data from five clinical trials of nesiritide administered by infusion for HF.

Most importantly, the drug is well-tolerated, simple, and safe to use when given in bolus/continuous–infusion fashion (2-μg/kg bolus followed by 0.01-μg/kg/min infusion) outside the ICU and without invasive hemodynamic monitoring. Tachyphylaxis does not seem to occur. The usual duration of infusion is approximately 24 to 48 hours, both in our experience and in the VMAC trial; however, more prolonged infusions may be used.

Hemodynamic Goals of Therapy

When attempting to tailor parenteral therapies using hemodynamic measurements, one should try to optimize systolic blood pressure. This is defined as the lowest pressure that adequately supports renal function and central nervous system activity without significant orthostatic symptoms (systolic blood pressure generally >80 to 90 mm Hg) (**Table 9.14**). Patient-specific hemodynamics usually include optimum filling pressure, which can be defined as the lowest pulmonary capillary wedge pressure (PCWP) that can be maintained without a preload-related decline in systolic blood pressure and/or cardiac index. A higher than normal PCWP (18 to 20 mm Hg) is sometimes required. Optimum afterload is the lowest systemic vascular resistance that leads to reasonable cardiac index while maintaining adequate systolic blood pressure (generally >80 mm Hg) and renal perfusion (generally urine output >0.5 cc/kg/hr).

Specific hemodynamic-directed protocols for decompensated HF therapy are summarized in **Table 9.15**.

TABLE 9.11 — HEMODYNAMIC EFFECTS OF PARENTERAL SUPPORT AGENTS USED IN DECOMPENSATED CONGESTIVE HEART FAILURE

Parenteral Agent	CO	HR	MAP	PCWP	PVR	SVR
Vasodilators						
Nesiritide (BNP)	↑	↔	↓↔	↓↓↓	↓	↓
Nitroglycerin	↑↓↔	↔	↓	↓↓	↓	↑
Nitroprusside	↑	↑	↓↓	↓	↓↓	↓
Phosphodiesterase Inhibitors						
Amrinone	↑	↑↔	↓↔	↓	↓	↓
Milrinone	↑	↑↔	↓↔	↓	↓	↓
Sympathomimetics						
Dobutamine	↑↑↑	↑↔	↓↔	↓↔	↓	↓
Dopamine, moderate dose (5-10 μg/kg/min)	↑↑	↑	↑↑	↑↔	↑	↑↔

Dopamine, high dose (>10 μg/kg/min)	↑	↑↑	↓↓	↑	↑↑	↑↑↑
Epinephrine	↑↑	↑↑↑	↑↔	↑↔	↑↑↑	→
Isoproterenol	↑↑↑	↑↑↑	↑↑	↓↓	→	↓↓
Norepinephrine	↓↑↔	↑↔↓	↑↑↑	↑↔	↑↑↑	↑↑↑
New Agents						
Levosimendan* (calcium sensitizer/PDEi)	↑↑	↑	→	→	→	→
Tezosentan (ERA)*	↑	↔	↓↔	→	→	→

Abbreviations: BNP, B-type natriuretic peptide; CO, cardiac output; ERA, endothelin receptor antagonist; HR, heart rate; MAP, mean arterial pressure; PCWP, pulmonary capillary wedge pressure; PDEi, phosphodiesterase inhibitor; PVR, pulmonary vascular resistance; SVR, systemic vascular resistance.

* Not yet approved for use.

TABLE 9.12 — SIDE EFFECTS OF AGENTS	
Side Effect	**Agent**
Arrhythmias	Dopamine, dobutamine, isoproterenol, epinephrine, norepinephrine, amirone, milrinone
Thiocyanate toxicity	Nitroprusside
Hypotension	All agents except dopamine, epinephrine, and norepinephrine
Excessive vasoconstriction	Norepinephrine, epinephrine, high-dose dopamine
Tachycardia	Dopamine, dobutamine, isoproterenol, epinephrine, norepinephrine
Thrombocytopenia	Amrinone

Nesiritide is the drug of choice when combined preload and afterload reduction is desired, and the most important goal is reduction of PCWP. Patients treated with nesiritide may be managed on a telemetry floor with routine noninvasive monitoring of cuff blood pressure. Nesiritide is usually started with a 2-µg/kg bolus followed by a 0.01-µg/kg/min infusion. However, many clinicians opt to start the standard-dose infusion without a loading bolus for a more gradual onset of vasodilation. Since the half-life of the drug is approximately 20 minutes, patients achieve steady state levels in $1^1/_2$ to 2 hours. Nesiritide should not be administered in the same intravenous (IV) infusion tubing as heparin or furosemide. The dose may be increased to 0.015 µg/kg/min, but further dose escalation above that dose is associated with more frequent hypotension and little incremental benefit.

Nitroglycerin and nesiritide have initially similar hemodynamic effects, but the very rapid onset of tachyphylaxis with nitroglycerin and the need for constant uptitration of dose make it a less attractive agent for HF

TABLE 9.13 — FIVE CLINICAL TRIALS OF NESIRITIDE IN HEART FAILURE

Author	No. of Subjects	Administration*	Results
Hobbs et al[130]	30	1, 3, 10, 15, 20 IV bolus	Hemodynamic improvement for 2-4 hours
Abraham et al[4]	16	0.025, 0.050 4-h IV infusion	Hemodynamic improvement during infusion
Mills et al[192]	103	0.015, 0.030, 0.060 24-h IV infusion	Hemodynamic improvement during infusion
Colucci et al[70]	127[†]	0.015 infusion	Hemodynamic improvement
	305[‡]	0.030 infusion	Improved clinical status
Publication Committee for the VMAC Investigators[244]	498	2.0 bolus; 0.010 infusion	Hemodynamic improvement; improved seven-point dyspnea scale; less diuretic use

Abbreviations: IV, intravenous; VMAC, Vasodilation in the Management of Acute Congestive Heart Failure.

* Dosages administered: µg/kg bolus; µg/kg/min infusion.

† Hemodynamic.

‡ Comparative.

Modified from: Mills RM, et al. *CHF*. 2002;8:270-273.

9

TABLE 9.14 — HEMODYNAMIC-DIRECTED PROTOCOLS FOR DECOMPENSATED HEART FAILURE THERAPY: HEMODYNAMIC GOALS

General Hemodynamic Goals
- Right atrial pressure 7 mm Hg
- PCWP 15 mm Hg
- SVR 1000 to 12000 dyne/sec/cm^5
- CI >2.5 1/min/m^2
- Optimum systolic or mean blood pressure is the lowest pressure that adequately supports renal function and central nervous system activity without significant orthostatic symptoms (systolic blood pressure generally >80 to 90 mm Hg)

Patient-Specific Hemodynamic Goals
- Optimum filling pressure (PCWP): lowest PCWP that can be maintained without preload-related decline in systolic blood pressure and/or CI. A higher PCWP (18 to 20 mm Hg) is usually required in acute myocardial injury
- Optimum afterload (SVR): lowest SVR that leads to reasonable CI while maintaining adequate systolic blood pressure (generally >80 mm Hg) and renal perfusion (urine output >0.5 cc/kg/h)

Abbreviations: CI, cardiac index; PCWP, pulmonary capillary wedge pressure; SVR, systemic vascular resistance.

management. The initial dose of nitroglycerin is usually 10 µg/min, and as much as 120 µg/min may be required to maintain an effect within a few hours.

Nitroprusside also produces combined preload and afterload reduction, and has been extensively studied in the tailored therapy approach to HF management. Treatment with nitroprusside requires admission to an ICU with invasive hemodynamic monitoring and experienced nursing staff; however, nitroprusside does offer the advantages of exquisitely sensitive dose titration and very rapid resolution of hemodynamic effects when discontinued. The starting dose is 0.1 to 0.2 µg/kg/min, with titration by 0.2-μg/kg/min increments as often as every 3 to 5 minutes.

Milrinone is generally used when cardiac output remains inadequate with optimal loading conditions and an inotrope is clinically indicated. In contrast to dobutamine, milrinone may be used in conjunction with β-blocker therapy. The dose range is 0.375 to 0.75 μg/kg/min and usually 0.5 μg/kg/min. As with other parenteral hemodynamic active agents, targets are desired cardiac pressures and flow. Excessive hypotension is often seen when using a loading dose. Generally, one can begin milrinone without loading, although this leads to a slight delay in onset of beneficial hemodynamic actions. Perhaps, in certain circumstances, milrinone is less arrhythmogenic than adrenergic agents, and some have suggested that it can be used more safely than dobutamine when HF and acute ischemic syndromes are apparent. The fact that milrinone can used in combination with β-blocker therapy is a potential advantage.

Dobutamine is chosen when both inotropic and vasodilating effects are desired, but inotropic effects are the most important. One should begin this agent at 2.5 μg/kg/min and attempt to keep the dose <10 to 15 μg/kg/min so that arrhythmias, including sinus tachycardia, are not noted. One might consider adding low-dose dopamine or milrinone to dobutamine in certain circumstances to augment further renal perfusion and/or achieve better hemodynamic end points. Hemodynamic effects resolve over minutes to hours when dobutamine and dopamine infusions are stopped, but benefits have been said to occasionally persist longer. β-Blockers will impair the response to dobutamine.

Table 9.16 summarizes the initial management of acute cardiogenic pulmonary edema and focuses on the importance of vasodilator therapy. This should be coupled with careful IV diuretic administration as well as supplemental O_2 and mechanical ventilation guided

**TABLE 9.15 — HEMODYNAMIC-DIRECTED
PROTOCOLS FOR DECOMPENSATED HEART
FAILURE THERAPY: SPECIFIC INTRAVENOUS
PHARMACOLOGIC THERAPY**

Nesiritide (vasodilator)

Begin when reduction of pulmonary capillary wedge and pulmonary artery pressures are the primary hemodynamic goal (most patients):

- May start with 2-µg/kg bolus followed by 0.01-µg/kg/min infusion, or start infusion without bolus if more gradual onset desired, ie, systolic blood pressure marginal for vasodilator therapy
- If needed, may increase infusion to 0.015 µg/kg/min
- Further dose escalation not usually associated with clinical benefit
- Onset of hemodynamic effects within 30 minutes after bolus + infusion, 90 minutes with infusion alone
- Binding and inactivation if infused via same tubing as heparin or furosemide
- No tachyphylaxis
- Hemodynamic effects dissipate rapidly when infusion stopped
- No arrhythmias noted
- Less diuretics required
- Enhanced natriuresis and diuresis

Milrinone ("inodilator")

Begin when both vasodilating and inotropic effects are desired; ie, persistent inadequate cardiac output after appropriate reductions in filling pressure and systemic vascular resistance:

- Dose range is 0.375 to 0.74 µg/kg/min (usual dose is 0.5 µg/kg/min)
- Target hemodynamic
- Excessive hypotension with loading dose; would avoid loading in acute heart failure
- Prolonged hemodynamic effects after drug is stopped
- Watch for arrhythmia

Dobutamine (inotrope)

Begin when inotropic effects are most important; do not use in patients receiving chronic β-blocker therapy:

- Start at 2.5 µg/kg/min
- Attempt to keep dose <15 µg/kg/min; avoid significant tachycardia
- May be more arrhythmogenic than milrinone (watch for occurrence)
- Consider adding low-dose dopamine or milrinone to assist in augmenting renal perfusion and/or achieving hemodynamic end points
- Hemodynamic effects resolve over minutes to hours when infusion is stopped, but benefits occasionally persist longer

Nitroglycerin (alternative vasodilator)

Begin when combined preload and afterload reduction is most important hemodynamic goal, but there is a greater desire to lower pulmonary capillary blood pressure than blood pressure.

- Start at 10 to 40 µg/min; difficult to pick best dose
- Titrate upward by 10 to 20 µg every 15 to 30 minutes until desired hemodynamics are reached
- May take >1 hour for best effects to be seen
- Tube/bag adsorption a problem
- Tachyphylaxis a problem; need to uptitrate dose regularly
- Hemodynamic effects resolve quickly when drug stopped

Nitroprusside (alternative vasodilator)

Begin when combined preload and afterload reduction is most important hemodynamic goal.

- Start at 0.1 to 0.2 µg/kg/min
- Titrate upward by 0.2 µg/kg/min at 3- to 5-minute intervals
- Target hemodynamic end points desired
- Need to have patient in ICU with arterial line most of the time
- Hemodynamic effects resolve rapidly when infusion stopped

9

TABLE 9.16— INITIAL MANAGEMENT OF ACUTE CARDIOGENIC PULMONARY EDEMA

- Nesiritide:
  - 2-µg/kg bolus followed by 0.010-µg/kg/min infusion; rarely need to uptitrate dose
- Nitroglycerin:
  - Sublingual: 0.4 mg every 5 minutes
  - Intravenous: start at 0.2 to 0.4 µg/kg/min
  - Uptitration required
- Furosemide (intravenous):
  - 20 to 40 mg initially or total of usual daily diuretic dose
  - Follow volume status closely
- Nitroprusside is an option but hemodynamic monitoring required
- Supplemental oxygen/mechanical ventilation as guided by arterial blood-gas analysis
- Consider intravenous morphine (2 to 6 mg) if no pulmonary contraindication
- Electrocardiogram/cardiac biomarkers to exclude myocardial infarction
- Echocardiogram to evaluate:
  - Ventricular function
  - Valvular status
  - Pericardium
- Proceed with urgent coronary angiography or reperfusion therapy if indicated
- Keep blood pressure under control

by arterial blood gas analysis. One should rapidly obtain an electrocardiogram and echocardiogram in such patients to determine if an acute ischemic syndrome is in progress and evaluate ventricular function, valve integrity, and status of the pericardium. If acute MI or an unstable coronary syndrome is present, one should consider proceeding toward urgent coronary angiography with percutaneous intervention and/or institution of reperfusion therapy should be planned.

When refractory HF rather than acutely decompensated CHF is present, one must reconsider the entire approach to a patient's problem (**Table 9.17**). Perhaps higher-risk operative procedures, such as coronary revascularization, mitral and aortic valve repair or replacement, LV aneurysmectomy, or other remodeling surgical procedures, would be helpful. Cardiac transplantation, as mentioned in the previous chapter, can be helpful in some situations. Not to be forgotten in patients with chronic refractory volume overload is dialysis or ultrafiltration, which can sometimes be quite helpful in controlling fluid. Occasionally, the use of chronic or intermittent parenteral drug infusions (eg, dobutamine, milrinone, nesiritide, diuretics) in the home environment is helpful as palliative care. There is no consensus about this, however, and few trials have been performed that can provide guidance. Finally, when the patient is terminal, hospice care can eliminate pain and suffering while giving psychological and spiritual support to the patient and the patient's family.

9

Figure 9.2 summarizes the approach to management of decompensated HF. Initial clinical and laboratory assessment should determine whether the patient can be managed at home or requires hospital admission. BNP levels offer useful adjunctive information in this decision. In our experience, patients with BNP levels >800 pg/mL will usually benefit from hospital admission. If the physician opts for home management, reassessment every 48 to 72 hours is prudent. If the patient does not respond promptly with subjective, objective, and laboratory improvement, including a return to his or her baseline compensated BNP levels, hospital admission should be urged.

Table 9.18 lists a series of recent reports documenting the efficacy of multidisciplinary outpatient HF management programs. An active outpatient HF management program reduces readmission and overall costs of care. The importance of coordinated management, with nurse practitioners, dietitians, social ser-

TABLE 9.17 — REFRACTORY HEART FAILURE TREATMENT OPTIONS*

Higher-Risk Operative Procedures
- Coronary revascularization
- Mitral valve repair/replacement
- Aortic valve repair/replacement
- Left ventricular aneurysmectomy
- Endoventricular patch reconstruction or infarct exclusion (Dor procedure)

Cardiac Transplantation
- Orthotopic
- Heterotopic (rarely)

Abandoned Operative Procedures
- Dynamic cardiomyoplasty
- Volume-reduction surgery (Batista procedure)
- Pericardiectomy

Chronic Dialysis (sometimes indicated)
- Peritoneal dialysis
- Hemofiltration
- Ultrafiltration

Hospice Care When Patient Terminal/Futile
- Eliminate pain and suffering with comfort care
- Psychological/spiritual support
- Family/caregiver support

Chronic/Intermittent Parenteral Drug Infusion
- Chronic home inotropes/inodilators for symptomatic relief (polarized opinions on this issue)

* Assuming that patients are aggressively managed with polypharmacy and that ancillary medical difficulties have been addressed adequately.

vices providers, and rehabilitation specialists in addition to physicians cannot be overemphasized.

The role of intermittent outpatient infusion of vasoactive drugs remains uncertain. The current American Heart Association (AHA)/American College of Cardiology (ACC) guidelines discourages intermittent

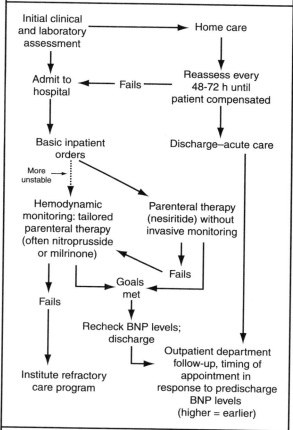

FIGURE 9.2 — DECOMPENSATED HEART FAILURE MANAGEMENT

Initial clinical and laboratory assessment → Home care

Home care → Reassess every 48-72 h until patient compensated

Reassess every 48-72 h until patient compensated → Fails → Admit to hospital

Initial clinical and laboratory assessment → Admit to hospital

Admit to hospital → Basic inpatient orders

Reassess every 48-72 h until patient compensated → Discharge–acute care

Basic inpatient orders → More unstable → Hemodynamic monitoring: tailored parenteral therapy (often nitroprusside or milrinone)

Basic inpatient orders → Parenteral therapy (nesiritide) without invasive monitoring

Parenteral therapy (nesiritide) without invasive monitoring → Fails → Hemodynamic monitoring: tailored parenteral therapy (often nitroprusside or milrinone)

Parenteral therapy (nesiritide) without invasive monitoring → Goals met

Hemodynamic monitoring: tailored parenteral therapy → Goals met

Hemodynamic monitoring: tailored parenteral therapy → Fails → Institute refractory care program

Goals met → Recheck BNP levels; discharge

Recheck BNP levels; discharge → Outpatient department follow-up, timing of appointment in response to predischarge BNP levels (higher = earlier)

Discharge–acute care → Outpatient department follow-up, timing of appointment in response to predischarge BNP levels (higher = earlier)

9

Abbreviation: BNP, B-type natriuretic peptide.

The management of an acutely decompensated congestive heart failure patient requires constant patient reassessment and delineation of goals.

TABLE 9.18 — MULTIDISCIPLINARY MANAGEMENT OF HEART FAILURE

Center	Publication Date	Intervention	No. of Subjects	Outcome
Washington University[249] St. Louis, Mo	November 1995	Nurse-directed, multidisciplinary	142 treated 140 controls	Improved survival, reduced readmissions, lower cost
UCLA[99] Los Angeles, Calif	September 1997	Comprehensive HF management program	214 before/after	Reduced readmissions, improved function, lower cost
Vanderbilt University[123] Nashville, Tenn	November 1997	Dedicated HF physicians	187 before/after	Reduced readmissions, increased volume
Midwest Heart[246] Lombard, Ill	January 1999	Multidisciplinary team	407 before 347 after	Reduced readmissions, lower cost
University of Adelaide[280] Australia	September 1999	Multidisciplinary team	100 treated 100 usual	Reduced readmissions, lower cost

Institution	Date	Program	Numbers	Outcomes
Duke University[306] Durham, NC	October 2001	Disease management program	117 treated before/after	Reduced hospitalization, lower cost
Yale University[157] New Haven, Conn	January 2002	Education/support	44 treated 44 controls	Reduced readmissions, lower cost
Johns-Hopkins[146] Baltimore, Md	February 2002	Multidisciplinary team	102 treated 98 controls	Reduced readmissions, fewer deaths
Gunderson Lutheran[7] LaCrosse, Wis	September 2002	HF clinic	38 treated 63 controls	Reduced readmissions

Abbreviation: HF, heart failure.

inotrope infusion; however, the recently completed Follow Up Serial Infusions of Nesiritide (FUSION) pilot trial suggests that intermittent outpatient infusions of nesiritide is safe and may benefit individuals refractory to standard oral agents[311] and has led to planning for a larger morbidity and mortality trial of this intervention.

10 Arrhythmia and Electrophysiologic Considerations

The hemodynamic, anatomic, and neurohormonal changes in clinical heart failure (HF) provide both the substrate for cardiac electrical dysfunction and heightened susceptibility to the adverse consequences of arrhythmia. State-of-the-art HF care requires a close working relationship between the HF clinician and the electrophysiologist. **Table 10.1** summarizes the electrophysiologic issues, and **Table 10.2**, the current controversies in the electrophysiology of HF. Many of these issues have been addressed in Chapter 3, *Pathophysiology*, and Chapter 6, *General Treatment Approaches*. This chapter will address nonpharmacologic, primarily device-oriented, approaches to three major electrophysiologic issues in HF:

- Asynchronous ventricular contraction due to electrical conduction delay (wide QRS)
- Atrial fibrillation (AF)
- Arrhythmogenic sudden death.

Pacing for Left Ventricular Dysfunction: Cardiac Resynchronization Therapy

Prolongation of the QRS duration >120 msec has been documented on routine electrocardiography in 20% to 50% of HF patients.[264] More ill populations generally have longer QRS delay. This degree of conduction delay produces asynchronous, mechanically ineffective, left ventricular (LV) contraction. There is a linear relationship between the degree of QRS prolon-

TABLE 10.1 — ELECTROPHYSIOLOGIC CONSIDERATIONS IN HEART FAILURE

- Prevalence of ventricular arrhythmias
- Prevalence of atrial arrhythmias
- Relationship of ventricular and atrial arrhythmias to worsening heart failure
- Relationship of ventricular and atrial arrhythmias to death
- Relationship of heart block and bradyarrhythmias to heart failure morbidity and mortality
- Pathophysiology of arrhythmias
- Best arrhythmia screening tactics
- Best therapeutic tactics

TABLE 10.2 — CONTROVERSIES IN ARRHYTHMIA MANAGEMENT IN HEART FAILURE

- Rate vs rhythm control in patients with atrial fibrillation
- Utility of routine arrhythmia screening in asymptomatic HF patients
- Safety of antiarrhythmic agents in HF patients
- Treatment of patients with asymptomatic, nonsustained ventricular tachycardia with antiarrhythmics or devices
- Indications for provocative EPS in LVD patients
- Implications of a positive EPS in LVD patients
- Indications for AICD implantation in LVD patients (prophylaxis vs treatment)
- Role of antibradycardia pacing in LVD patients
- Best physiologic pacing strategies in LVD patients
- Role of biventricular cardiac resynchronization pacing in LVD patients

Abbreviation: AICD, automatic implantable cardioverter defibrillator; EPS, electrophysiologic study; HF, heart failure; LVD, left ventricular dysfunction.

gation and decreases in ejection fraction (EF), and QRS prolongation is a marker for increased mortality in HF. With the development of LV pacing leads placed either directly or by way of the coronary sinus and pulse generators capable of biventricular pacing, pacemaker therapy for cardiac resynchronization (CRT) has become a practical approach to this problem (**Figure 10.1** and **Figure 10.2**).[161] **Table 10.3** summarizes the available clinical trial data supporting the efficacy of this approach.

In our opinion, the evidence supporting the benefits of cardiac resynchronization therapy (CRT) in HF is conclusive, with documented improvement in quality of life, New York Heart Association (NYHA) functional class, and 6-minute walk performance, as well as neurohormonal improvement. Nonetheless, a number of questions remain:

- Where should the QRS threshold be set?
- What should constitute optimal clinical, laboratory, and functional indications for CRT? Should asymptomatic or minimally symptomatic individuals receive devices to prevent progression to more severe HF?
- What are the indications for CRT in AF?
- Should implantable cardioverter defibrillator (ICD) capabilities be standard in these devices?

We look forward to future clinical trials to provide more evidence-based answers to these questions. **Figure 10.3** presents an algorithm that outlines our current practice. In addition, we recommend placement of LV epicardial leads for patients with an EF <30%, CHF, and QRS duration >120 msec who are undergoing cardiac surgery in order to facilitate resynchronization pacing postoperatively, if needed. Leads can be buried subcutaneously and used at a later date. Though successful percutaneous insertion of CRT de-

**FIGURE 10.1 — RESYNCHRONIZATION
THERAPY IN HEART FAILURE**

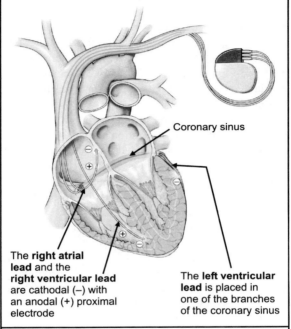

Coronary sinus

The **right atrial
lead** and the
right ventricular lead
are cathodal (–) with
an anodal (+) proximal
electrode

The **left ventricular
lead** is placed in
one of the branches
of the coronary sinus

Many patients with congestive heart failure might benefit from a new type of pacemaker capable of cardiac
resynchronization by correcting delays in conduction that
result in different regions of the heart when the QRS is
>120 msec.

Adapted from: Khaykin Y, et al. *Cleve Clin J Med.* 2003;70:
853.

vices is now 90% to 95%, some patients with failures
of insertion or suboptimal placement of pacing cath-
eters can go for mini-thoracotomy or thorascopic insertion operations.

FIGURE 10.2 — RETROGRADE CORONARY SINUS ANGIOGRAM

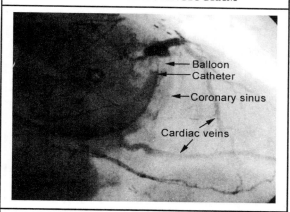

Retrograde coronary sinus angiogram in the anteroposterior projection using a balloon-tip catheter. After cannulation, the balloon is inflated to occlude the main coronary sinus, allowing for better retrograde filling of the venous branches and helping guide LV lead placement.

Adapted from: Khaykin Y, et al. *Cleve Clin J Med.* 2003;70: 853.

Atrial Fibrillation

Atrial fibrillation affects an estimated 2.2 million adults in the United States, and by virtue of numbers poses the greatest arrhythmia management challenge in HF care. **Table 10.4** and **Figure 10.4** outline the classification of AF and the magnitude of the challenge in the coming years. **Table 10.5** lists a number of conditions that predispose patients to AF. Although not usually acutely life-threatening, this arrhythmia is far from benign. The physiologic effects of AF include:

- Loss of atrial contribution to ventricular filling
- Lack of rate control associated with variable diastolic filling

261

TABLE 10.3 — RANDOMIZED CLINICAL TRIALS OF BIVENTRICULAR CARDIAC RESYNCHRONIZATION PACING

Study	N	Inclusion Criteria	Main Results, Comments
PATH-CHF*[18-20]	41	NYHA class 3 or 4 QRS >120 ms PR >150 ms Sinus rate >55	Improved hemodynamics (LV pacing had better acute hemodynamic results than CRT) Improved $Vo_{2\ max}$ Improved 6-minute walking distance
MUSTIC[55,162,169]	58	NYHA class 3 QRS >150 ms EF ≤35% LVEDD >60 mm No pacing indications	Improved exercise capacity and quality of life Fewer hospitalizations for CHF 85% of patients preferred CRT Not designed to assess mortality, but showed a 5% reduction in mortality at 6 months, all in biventricular-paced patients
MIRACLE[2,3,75,281]	453	NYHA class 3 or 4 QRS ≥130 ms EF ≤35% LVEDD ≥55 mm No pacing indications Stable medical regimen	Improved NYHA class Improved 6-minute walking distance Improved quality of life Small improvement in EF About 2/3 of patients classified as improved, but 39% also improved despite no pacing therapy (placebo effect)

		Fewer CHF hospitalizations Improved end systolic volume Improved end diastolic volume Reduced mitral regurgitation
MIRACLE ICD[168,282,308]	369	No standard indications for ICD	Improved NYHA class Improved peak $VO_{2\,max}$ Improved quality of life Evaluated CRT in patients with CHF who needed an ICD without interference of device function
		NYHA class 3–4 QRS ≥130 ms EF ≤35% No pacing indications Standard ICD indications	
MIRACLE ICD II[313]	210	NYHA class 2 QRS >130 ms EF <35% No pacing indications Standard ICD indications	Improved clinical composite response Improved echocardiogram, but primary end point ($VO_{2\,max}$) not changed Improved EF
Contak CD[80]	490	NYHA class 2–4 QRS ≥120 ms EF ≤35% Standard ICD indications	Decreased progression of CHF (21%), but did not achieve the prespecified 25% reduction Improved $VO_{2\,max}$ in NYHA class 3 and 4 Improved 6-minute walking distance in NYHA class 3 and 4 Improved quality of life in NYHA class 3 and 4

Continued

10

Study	N	Inclusion Criteria	Main Results, Comments
COMPANION[38]	1520	NYHA class 3 or 4 QRS ≥120 ms EF ≤35% No standard indications for pacing or ICD Stable medical regimen	Stopped due to lower mortality and hospitalization rates First controlled study to include a mortality end point Uses over-the-wire pacing system
InSync III[145,165]	264	NYHA class 3 or 4 QRS ≥130 ms EF ≤35% LVEDD ≥55 mm No pacing indications	Improved NYHA, quality of life, exercise capacity compared with historic MIRACLE study control Device allows for differential ventricular pacing and programmable V-V interval Uses over-the-wire pacing system
Vector	—	NYHA class 2–4 QRS ≥140 ms EF ≤35% LVEDD ≥55 mm	Ongoing
CARE-HF[323]	814	NYHA class 3 or 4 QRS ≥120 ms EF ≤35% No pacing or standard ICD indication	Ongoing Highest powered study with longest follow-up to assess effect of CRT on morbidity and hospitalization

Abbreviations: CARE-HF, Cardiac Resynchronization in Heart Failure; CHF, congestive heart failure; COMPANION, Comparison of Medical Therapy, Pacing and Defibrillation in Chronic Heart Failure; CRT, cardiac resynchronization therapy; EF, ejection fraction; ICD, implantable cardioverter-defibrillator; LV, left ventricular; LVEDD, left ventricular end-diastolic dimensions; MIRACLE, Multicenter InSync Randomized Clinic Evaluation; MIRACLE ICD, Multicenter InSync Randomized Clinic Evaluation Implantable Cardioverter Defibrillator; MUSTIC, Multisite Stimulation in Cardiomyopathy; NYHA, New York Heart Association; PATH-CHF, Pacing Therapies for Congestive Heart Failure; $Vo_{2\,max}$, peak oxygen consumption.

* Crossover trials.

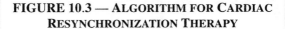

FIGURE 10.3 — ALGORITHM FOR CARDIAC
RESYNCHRONIZATION THERAPY

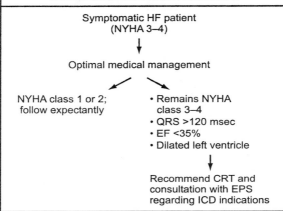

Abbreviations: CRT; cardiac resynchronization therapy;
EF, ejection fraction; EPS, electrophysiology study; HF,
heart failure; ICD, implantable cardioverter defibrillator;
NYHA, New York Heart Association.

- Tachycardia contributing to further left ventricular dysfunction (LVD)
- Lack of appropriate rate response to exercise.

Figure 10.5 summarizes management strategies for
cardioversion of AF lasting >48 hours. Cardioversion
can be accomplished either electrically or pharmacologically. Often, a combination of the two is used. The
duration of AF is directly related to the risk of embolic stroke during cardioversion. Common practice dictates that patients in continuous AF for >48 hours
should receive warfarin for 3 to 6 weeks before
cardioversion in order to decrease the risk of embolic
stroke as atrial function is returned, regardless of the
method of cardioversion. Transesophageal echocardiography can provide an alternative approach as outlined in **Figure 10.5**. Cardioversion of AF of unknown

TABLE 10.4 — BASIC CLASSIFICATION OF THE TYPES OF ATRIAL FIBRILLATION

Type of AF	Classification
Lone	Occurs in the absence of cardiac or other conditions predisposing to AF
Acute	Generally refers to AF lasting <48 hours
Paroxysmal	Generally is characterized by recurrent, transient episodes that revert to sinus rhythm spontaneously or with treatment
Persistent	Does not convert to sinus rhythm without intervention or cardioversion
Permanent AF	Persistent despite cardioversion
Abbreviation: AF, atrial fibrillation.	
Adapted from: Chung MK. *Cleve Clin J Med.* 2003;70:S7.	

duration with transesophageal echocardiographic guidance, in conjunction with short-term anticoagulation, seems as safe as conventional therapy and minimizes the total duration of anticoagulation, AF, and atrial mechanical dysfunction.

Table 10.6 lists the antiarrhythmic drugs that have been used to convert or control AF in the modified Vaughan-Williams classification scheme. Chemical cardioversion can be attempted with any of the class 1A, 1C, and 3 antiarrhythmic drugs; however, in patients with systolic LVD and HF, class 1 antiarrhythmic drugs are associated with detrimental effects when given long-term. The Cardiac Arrhythmia Suppression Trial (CAST) used class 1C antiarrhythmic agents (flecainide, encainide, and propafenone) in patients with premature ventricular contractions post–myocardial infarction.[51-53,119] This study demonstrated a high mortality in patients treated with drugs compared with

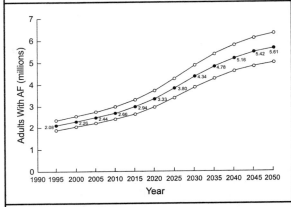

FIGURE 10.4 — PROJECTED NUMBER OF ADULTS WITH ATRIAL FIBRILLATION IN THE UNITED STATES, 1995 TO 2050

Abbreviation: AF, atrial fibrillation.

Upper and lower curves represent the upper and lower projections based on sensitivity analysis.

Adapted from: Go AS, et al. *JAMA*. 2001;285:2370-2375.

placebo, although this was not an AF trial. Class 3 drugs (sotalol and amiodarone) are safest for patients with significant systolic LVD.[12,56,175,237,268,269,271] Sotalol should be avoided in patients with renal failure, and it has β-blocking effects that could prove problematic in patients with bronchospastic disease, severely impaired LV function, or in whom other β-blockers have been prescribed. Careful monitoring of the QT interval is essential in patients taking sotalol. When amiodarone is used for AF, an initial loading dose of 600 mg daily for 1 month followed by 200 mg daily is usually effective. Adverse events occur frequently and include:

- Pulmonary fibrosis
- Hypothyroidism and thyrotoxicosis
- Hepatic dysfunction

TABLE 10.5 — CONDITIONS AND FACTORS THAT CAN PREDISPOSE TO ATRIAL FIBRILLATION

- Hypertension
- Ischemic heart disease
- Advanced age
- Rheumatic heart disease*
- Nonrheumatic valve disease
- Cardiomyopathies
- Congestive heart failure
- Congenital heart disease
- Sick sinus syndrome/degenerative conduction system disease
- Wolff-Parkinson-White syndrome
- Pericarditis
- Pulmonary embolism
- Thyrotoxicosis
- Chronic lung disease
- Neoplastic disease
- Diabetes
- Postoperative state

* Especially mitral valve disease.

Adapted from: Chung MK. *Cleve Clin J Med.* 2003;70:S8.

10

- Lenticular opacities
- A bluish discoloration of the skin.

Thyroid, liver, and pulmonary function studies should be obtained every 6 months, and a yearly ophthalmologic examination should be performed in patients on chronic amiodarone. Drugs that slow conduction across the atrioventricular node (AVN), such as digoxin, diltiazem, verapamil, and β-blockers, can be helpful in attenuating the ventricular response to AF but do not result in conversion to sinus rhythm. Although useful in the acute management of AF to slow the ventricular rate and stabilize hemodynamics, AVN blockers are not essential to a cardioversion strategy.

FIGURE 10.5 — MANAGEMENT OF ATRIAL FIBRILLATION LASTING >48 HOURS IN HEART FAILURE PATIENTS

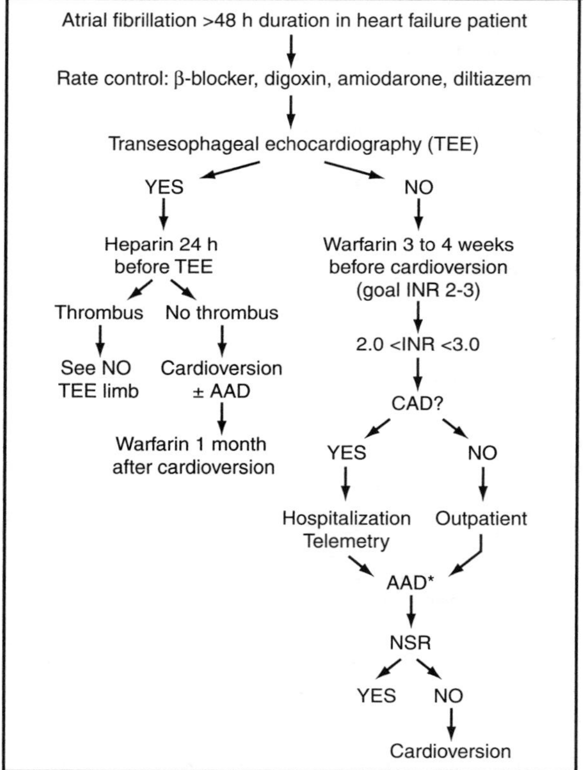

Atrial fibrillation >48 h duration in heart failure patient

↓

Rate control: β-blocker, digoxin, amiodarone, diltiazem

↓

Transesophageal echocardiography (TEE)

YES ← → NO

YES:
Heparin 24 h before TEE
→ Thrombus / No thrombus

Thrombus → See NO TEE limb

No thrombus → Cardioversion ± AAD → Warfarin 1 month after cardioversion

NO:
Warfarin 3 to 4 weeks before cardioversion (goal INR 2-3)

↓

2.0 <INR <3.0

↓

CAD?

YES → Hospitalization Telemetry

NO → Outpatient

→ AAD*

↓

NSR

YES / NO

NO → Cardioversion

Abbreviations: AAD, antiarrhythmic drug; CAD, coronary artery disease; INR, international normalized ratio; NSR, normal sinus rhythm.

* When ejection fraction (EF) <40%, use amiodarone only. When EF >40%, use sotalol or amiodarone in hospitalized CAD patients. May consider vascular wall class IA, IC, III AAD in patients with EF >40% and no CAD.

Modifed from: Conti JB. Management of atrial fibrillation. In: Mills RM, Young JB, eds. *Practical Approaches to the Treatment of Heart Failure*. Baltimore, Md: Williams and Wilkins; 1998.

TABLE 10.6 — ANTIARRHYTHMIC DRUGS USED TO TREAT ATRIAL FIBRILLATION

Class IA Agents
- Disopyramide (Norpace and others)
- Procainamide (Procanbid and others)
- Quinidine (Quinidex and others)

Class IC Agents
- Flecainide (Tambocor)
- Propafenone (Rythmol)
- Moricizine (Ethmozine)

Class II Agents
- β-Blockers (eg, metoprolol)

Class III Agents
- Amiodarone (Cordarone and others)
- Dofetilide (Tikosyn)
- Ibutilide (Corvert)
- Sotalol (Betapace AF)

Class IV Agents
- Calcium channel blockers (eg, verapamil, diltiazem)

Adapted from: Martin DO, et al. *Cleve Clin J Med.* 2003;70: S13.

10

Antiarrhythmic medications administered to achieve known therapeutic drug concentration levels appear to facilitate electrical cardioversion. Electrical cardioversion requires short-acting general anesthesia. For a synchronized, direct current cardioversion, an initial energy setting of 200 joules is recommended, followed by 300 and then 360 joules, if needed.

Early conversion of AF may help to avoid the electrical and physical changes in the atria that predispose to recurrent and/or sustained AF, and maintenance of sinus rhythm may, in fact, reverse electrical remodeling. However, in the AFFIRM trial, the largest trial to date comparing rate-control to rhythm-control management strategies, no survival benefit or quality-of-life improvement was achieved with rhythm control.

For patients with refractory rapid response to AF, AVN ablation with implantation of a permanent pacemaker can improve symptoms, quality of life, and LVD due to chronic tachycardia. A meta-analysis of 21 small studies totaled 1181 patients who improved in 18 of 19 outcome measures.[308] Anticoagulation, of course, must be continued. The other disadvantages to this approach include pacemaker dependence and the possible need for CRT in some patients as atrial-ventricular pacing alone has been noted to be detrimental in HF (DAVID trial).[307]

Pacemaker therapy may also play an important adjunctive role in management of paroxysmal AF in patients who require pacing for standard indications, usually sick sinus syndrome. **Table 10.7** lists a series of trials of algorithm-based pacing to prevent AF. Variations in the patient populations and pacing protocols complicate interpretation, but it appears that if almost constant atrial pacing can be achieved, the pacing protocols may be effective.

For AF patients who are candidates for surgical intervention of structural heart disease, and for some selected individuals with symptomatic AF in whom conventional therapies have failed, surgical management offers an effective option. In the Cleveland Clinic experience, Maze surgery for AF is performed most frequently in conjunction with other procedures. In 2001 (the most recent complete data set), 37% of AF surgeries were for lone AF, whereas 27% were done with mitral valve repair, 11% with mitral valve replacement, 11% with coronary bypass grafting, and 14% with other procedures. Overall operative mortality was 1.9%, and approximately 95% were free of AF at 6 months postsurgery.[185]

Many refractory AF patients, however, do not have indications for cardiac surgery. Patients with symptomatic, drug-refractory AF should be offered consideration for catheter-based pulmonary vein isolation.

Table 10.8 presents a summary of the large published series of catheter-based ablation studies. The highest success rates with the lowest complication rates are produced with empiric circumferential pulmonary vein isolation guided by intracardiac echocardiography. Catheter ablation is safe and effective for most patients; catheter technology and operator experience are critical for success. Complications, including pulmonary vein stenosis, occur with a relatively low incidence; however, patient selection must weigh risk vs benefit, and good communication between the HF clinician and the electrophysiologist is critically important.

As **Figure 10.6** emphasizes, the options for effective management of AF today have expanded far beyond digoxin and warfarin. Dramatic responses to nonpharmacologic management, often combined with optimal pharmacotherapy as well, mean that many HF patients with AF can look forward to improved functional capacity with surgery, ablation therapy, or pacing.

Ventricular Arrhythmias and Prevention of Sudden Cardiac Death

Sudden cardiac death (SCD) refers to death that occurs within an hour of the onset of symptoms from an unexpected circulatory arrest. The phenomenon of SCD usually represents the pathophysiologic effects of ventricular arrhythmia in the setting of advanced structural heart disease. Estimates of the frequency of SCD in the HF population vary from roughly 25% to 50%[64,66,128,271,276]; sustained monomorphic ventricular tachycardia probably leads to most of these deaths. HF patients with unexplained syncope should be considered at particularly high risk for subsequent SCD.[194]

Based on the huge number of HF patients and their high risk of SCD, attempts to develop an evidence-based approach to arrhythmia management have led to **a number of clinical trials.** As the discipline of large-

					Length of	

TABLE 10.7 — SELECTED TRIALS OF ALGORITHM-BASED PACING TO PREVENT ATRIAL FIBRILLATION

Study/ Investigators	N	Study Design	Pacing Mode/Site	Pacing Algorithm(s)	Length of Follow-Up (months)	Reduction in AF Burden
Padeletti et al[219]	46	R, P, CO	DDDR; IAS or RAA	CAP on vs off	6	Not significant
AT500[136]	325	L, P	DDDR	3 algorithms* on + ATP	3	Not significant
ADOPT-A[54]	288	R, P	DDDR 60 bpm	DAO on vs off	6	25%
AFT (phase 3)[135]	92	R, P	DDD 70 bpm	4 algorithms† on vs off	2	30%
ASPECT[220]	294	R, P, CO	DDDR; IAS or RAA	3 algorithms* on vs off	6	Not significant
ATTEST[163]	370	R, P	DDDR	3 algorithms* on vs off ± ATP	3	Not significant
PIPAF 2[258]	44	R, P, CO	Dual-site DDD 70 bpm	SRO on vs off	6	Not significant
PIPAF 4[258]	47	R, P, CO	DDDR 70 bpm	SRO on vs off	6	Not significant

Abbreviations: ADOPT-A, Atrial Dynamic Overdrive Pacing Trial; AFT, Atrial Fibrillation Therapy [trial]; ASPECT, Atrial Septal Pacing Efficacy Clinical Trial; ATP, atrial antitachycardia pacing; ATTEST, Atrial Therapy Efficacy and Safety Trial; bpm, beats per minute; CAP, consistent atrial pacing; CO, crossover; DAO, dynamic atrial overdrive; DDD, dual chamber pacing–no rate modulation or multisite pacing; DDDR, dual chamber, adaptive-rate pacing–no multisite pacing; IAS, interatrial septum; L, longitudinal; P, prospective; PIPAF, Pacing in Prevention of Atrial Fibrillation; R, randomized; RAA, right atrial appendage; SRO, sinus rhythm overdrive.

* Atrial preference pacing, atrial rate stabilization, and postmode switch overdrive pacing.
† Premature atrial complex (PAC) suppression, postexercise response, atrial overdrive pacing, and post-PAC response.

Adapted from: Martin DO, et al. *Cleve Clin J Med.* 2003;70:S18.

10

TABLE 10.8 — SUMMARY OF LARGE PUBLISHED SERIES OF CATHETER-BASED ABLATION FOR ATRIAL FIBRILLATION

Study	Technique	Imaging	No. PVs Targeted	N	Cured (%)	Complications (no. or %)	Follow-Up (months)	Length of Procedure
Haissaguerre, 1996[115]	Maze	F	NA	45	22	Atrial flutter (19), hemopericardium (1)	11 ± 4	248 ± 79 min
Haissaguerre, 1998[116]	FA	F	Active	45	62	None	8 ± 6	NA
Chen, 1999[59]	FA	F	Active	79	86	PV stenosis (42%), CVA (2), hemothorax (1), hemopericardium (1)	6 ± 2	90 ± 32 min
Gerstenfeld, 2001[103]	FA, CA	F	Active	71	23	PV stenosis (8.3%)	60 ± 33	7.5 ± 2 hr
Sanders, 2002[257]	FA	F	Active	51	30	PV stenosis (1)	11 ± 8	NA
Natale, 2000[202]	CA	F, US	2 superior + LIPV	15	60	CVA (1)	7 ± 2	224 ± 89 min
Saliba, 2002[256]	CA	F, US	2 superior + active	33	39	CVA (1), PV stenosis (1)	29 ± 6	224 ± 89 min
Pappone, 2000[224]	CA	F, C	4	26	62	None	9 ± 3	370 ± 58 min
Pappone, 2001[223]	CA	F, C	4	251	75	Tamponade (2)	10 ± 4.5	148 ± 26 min

Haissaguerre, 2000[114]	CA	F	Active	90	71	PV stenosis	8 ± 5	278 ± 154 min
Haissaguerre, 2000[117]	CA	F	Active	70	73	None	4 ± 5	206 ± 49 min
Kanagaratnam, 2001[144]	CA	F, C	2 superior + active	71	21	Flutter (20%), PV stenosis (17%)	29 ± 8	365 ± 77 min
Oral, 2002[205]	CA	F	2 superior, 1 inferior	70	70 parox, 22 persist	Retinal embolus (1)	5	NA
Mangrum, 2002[179]	CA	F, ICE	Active	56	66	CVA (3), tamponade (1)	13 ± 7	243 ± 75 min
Oral, 2002[204]	CA	F	2–3	40	85	None	148 ± 87 days	277 ± 59 min
Macle, 2002[173]	CA	F	4	136	66	None	8 ± 5	188 ± 54 min
Marrouche, 2002[181]	FA CA	F F, 4 mm F, 8 mm F, cooled	Active 4 4 4	21 47 21 122	29 79 100 85	PV stenosis (3) PV stenosis (1), CVA (1) None PV stenosis (1), CVA (1), tamponade (2)	11 ± 3 10 ± 3 8 ± 4 4 ± 2	5.4 ± 3 hr 5.5 ± 3 hr 3 ± 1 hr 4 ± 1 hr

Continued

Study	Technique	Imaging	No. PVs Targeted	N	Cured (%)	Complications (no. or %)	Follow-Up (months)	Length of Procedure
Marrouche, 2003[182]	CA	F	4	56	80	PV stenosis (3), embolic event (2)	417 ± 145 days	250 ± 66 min
		F, ICE	4	107	83	PV stenosis (2), embolic event (3)	417 ± 145 days	190 ± 48 min
		F, ICE, MB	4	152	90	None	417 ± 145 days	185 ± 65 min
Chen, 2002[58] (substudy, EF <45%)	CA	F, ICE, MB	4	30	70	Pulmonary edema (3%), CVA (3%)	12 ± 5	NA
Deisenhofer, 2003[83]	CA	F	3	75	51	PV stenosis (6)	230 ± 133 days	353 ± 143 min

Abbreviations: C, CARTO mapping; CA, circumferential ablation; cooled, catheter with cooled tip; CVA, cerebrovascular accident; EF, ejection fraction; F, fluoroscopy; FA, focal ablation; ICE, intracardiac echocardiography; LIPV, left inferior pulmonary vein; MB, microbubbles; NA, not available; parox, paroxysmal atrial fibrillation; persist, persistent atrial fibrillation; PV, pulmonary vein; US, balloon-tipped ultrasound catheter; 4 mm, catheter with 4-mm tip; 8 mm, catheter with 8-mm tip.

Adapted from: Martin DO, et al. *Cleve Clin J Med.* 2003;70:S25.

FIGURE 10.6 — MANAGEMENT OF ATRIAL FIBRILLATION WHEN CARDIOVERSION FAILS IN HEART FAILURE PATIENTS

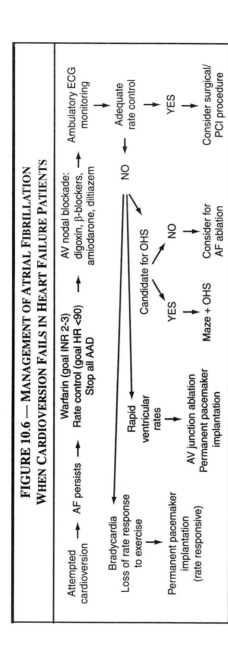

Abbreviations: AAD, antiarrhythmic drug; AF, atrial fibrillation; AV, atrioventricular; ECG, electrocardiogram; HR, heart rate (beats/min); INR, international normalized ratio; OHS, open-heart surgery; PCI, percutaneous coronary intervention.

Modified from: Conti JB. Management of atrial fibrillation. In: Mills RM, Young JB, eds. *Practical Approaches to the Treatment of Heart Failure*. Baltimore, Md: Williams and Wilkins; 1998.

scale clinical trials in HF has developed over the past quarter-century, investigators have learned that studying as-yet-unproven therapies in the highest risk populations initially yields meaningful results most ethically and efficiently. Following this principle, the initial trials comparing ICD efficacy vs pharmacologic management were secondary prevention trials, enrolling patients who had survived an episode of SCD or life-threatening arrhythmia. **Table 10.9** summarizes four major multicenter international secondary prevention trials. The AVID trial, which was by far the largest of the four, was terminated early because of significant ICD benefit.

The impact of the secondary prevention data prompted a number of primary prevention trials in high-risk populations. We have data from four published trials and one preliminary report from a completed but as-yet unpublished trial. Several more studies are ongoing. **Table 10.10** summarizes the primary prevention trial data. The MADIT II findings suggest that for coronary disease patients, risk stratification on the basis of EF may be as effective as invasive electrophysiologic testing. The SCD-HeFT findings have been reported but not yet formally reviewed and published.[324] SCD-Heft included 2521 NYHA II-III subjects with EF ≤35%, with or without coronary disease. Patients were on optimal medical therapy for HF and were randomized in equal numbers to placebo (n = 847), amiodarone (n = 845), and an implantable defibrillator programmed for ventricular fibrillation therapy only (n = 829). Overall, ICD subjects had a highly significant reduction in all-cause mortality, 23% compared with placebo. On intention-to-treat analysis, amiodarone was not associated with any improvement in mortality compared with placebo. These findings have very significant implications for clinical care and medical economics.

In aggregate, the data from these trials now require that clinicians who care for HF patients view all NYHA Class II or higher patients with systolic LVD and EF ≤35% as at risk for SCD and as having a valid indication for ICD therapy. Unfortunately, insurers (primarily the federal government), clinical trialists, and practitioners will have to come to a consensus on how to deal with the implications of this new approach to arrhythmia management. **Table 10.11** outlines indications for electrophysiologic study in HF patients, and **Figure 10.7** presents our recommendations for management of SCD survivors. Many HF patients show nonsustained ventricular tachycardia (NSVT) on routine monitoring or on exercise testing. **Figure 10.8** outlines our approach to NSVT.

■ The Biventricular Pacer-Defibrillator

As device technology has progressed, the prospect of employing a more complete electrophysiologic approach to HF management with a device capable of biventricular pacing and defibrillation has evolved. **Table 10.12** lists some of the ongoing trials that are likely to provide evidence to guide future management strategies at the interface of electrophysiology and HF. **Figure 10.9** illustrates a proposed algorithm for integrating the biventricular pacemaker-defibrillator into current management.

Devices have drawbacks. Current concerns include the duration of the implantation procedure, which may require $2^{1}/_{2}$ to 3 hours for biventricular pacemakers. Complications include:
- Coronary sinus dissection
- Perforation
- Failure to implant the device successfully
- Death (rarely).

TABLE 10.9 — MAJOR MULTICENTER INTERNATIONAL SECONDARY PREVENTION TRIALS OF SUDDEN CARDIAC DEATH

Trial	N	Entry Criteria	Primary End Point	LVEF (Mean %)	Outcome
AVID[14]	1016	VF arrest; syncope VT; VT with LVEF <40	All-cause mortality: drugs vs device	31 (drugs) 32 (device)	Terminated early due to significant ICD benefit
CIDS[72]	659	VT >150 bpm; inducible VT after unmonitored syncope	All-cause mortality; arrythmic death; amiodarone vs device	≤35	Decreased mortality and arrhythmic death with ICD, but *not* statistically significant
CASH[158]	349	SCD survivors	Mortality: propafenone vs amiodarone/metoprolol vs device	46	Borderline significant reduction (23%, $P = 0.08$) with ICD

			Mortality: drugs vs device		Significant mortality reduction with device
Wever et al[305]	60	VT/VF survivors with CAD and inducible VT		29 (drugs) 30 (device)	

Abbreviations: AVID, Antiarrhythmic vs Implantable Defibrillator [trial]; bpm, beats per minute; CAD, coronary artery disease; CASH, Cardiac Arrest Study Hamburg; CIDS, Canadian Implantable Defibrillator Study; ICD, implantable cardioverter defibrillator; LVEF, left ventricular ejection fraction; SCD, sudden cardiac death; VF, ventricular fibrillation; VT, ventricular tachycardia.

10

TABLE 10.10 — SUDDEN CARDIAC DEATH: MAJOR PRIMARY PREVENTION TRIALS				
Trial	N	Entry Criteria	Primary End Point	Outcome
MADIT[198]	196 (101: drug) (95: device)	Q-wave MI; LVEF ≤35%; NSVT; inducible VT	Drugs vs device; all-cause mortality	Premature termination due to mortality reduction with ICD
CABG Patch[34]	900 (446: device) (454: control)	CAD (CABG); LVEF <36%; abnormal SAECG	Mortality	No device benefit; SAECG inferior to EPS for risk stratification
MUSTT[45]	2202 65% noninducible registry; 35% inducible	Prior MI; LVEF ≤40%; NSVT	Mortality; ICD vs no therapy vs AAD	Mortality: ICD = 24%, no therapy = 48%, AAD = 55% SCD: ICD = 9%, no ICD = 37%
MADIT II[199]	1232 (490: drug) (742: device)	Prior MI; LVEF ≤30%	All-cause mortality	31% Risk reduction with ICD
SCD-HeFT[324]	2521 (847: placebo) (845: drug) (829: device)	NYHA II-III, with or without CAD, LVEF ≤35%	All-cause mortality	23% Risk reduction with ICD

Abbreviations: AAD, antiarrhythmic drug; CABG, coronary artery bypass graft; CAD, coronary artery disease; EPS, extrapyramidal symptom; ICD, implantable cardioverter defibrillator; LVEF, left ventricular ejection fraction; MADIT, Multicenter Automatic Defibrillator Implantation Trial; MI, myocardial infarction; MUSTT, Multicenter Unstable Tachycardia Trial; NSVT, nonsustained ventricular tachycardia; SAECG, signal-averaged electrocardiogram; SCD, sudden cardiac death; VT, ventricular tachycardia.

10

**TABLE 10.11 — INDICATIONS FOR
ELECTROPHYSIOLOGIC STUDY OF
VENTRICULAR ARRHYTHMIAS
IN HEART FAILURE PATIENTS**

Problems
- Cardiac arrest
- Sustained ventricular tachycardia with symptoms/syncope
- Wide complex tachycardia of uncertain cause (particularly when rapid or sustained)
- Syncope without noncardiac reason
- Nonsustained ventricular tachycardia and coronary artery disease with LVEF <35%

Therapy
- Appropriate device implantation

Abbreviation: LVEF, left ventricular ejection fraction.

In addition, infection occurs in up to 1.5% of biventricular implants, probably related to longer procedures. Given the costs and risks of device therapy, continued clinical research to refine the indications, risks, and benefits of this therapy will be required. However, it is quite evident now that these devices substantially improve the quality and length of life for select CHF patients. One of the most critical questions will involve whether a strategy of treating all those at risk on the basis of systolic dysfunction is superior to a targeted approach using multifactorial risk predictors, including anatomic, imaging, electrophysiologic study, and neurohormonal markers. As with creation of a multidrug protocol or in referral for surgical intervention, patient selection is critical.

FIGURE 10.7 — MANAGEMENT OF PATIENTS AFTER CARDIAC ARREST

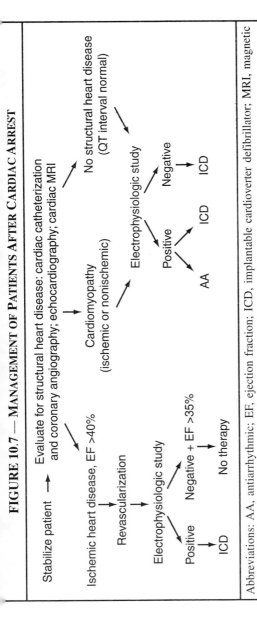

Abbreviations: AA, antiarrhythmic; EF, ejection fraction; ICD, implantable cardioverter defibrillator; MRI, magnetic resonance imaging.

Modified from: Curtis AB. Management of the patient at risk for sudden cardiac death. In: Mills RM, Young JB, eds. *Practical Approaches to the Treatment of Heart Failure.* Baltimore, Md: Williams and Wilkins; 1998.

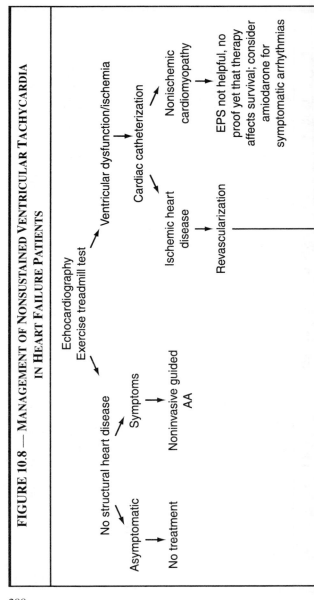

FIGURE 10.8 — MANAGEMENT OF NONSUSTAINED VENTRICULAR TACHYCARDIA IN HEART FAILURE PATIENTS

Echocardiography
Exercise treadmill test

No structural heart disease → Ventricular dysfunction/ischemia

Asymptomatic → No treatment

Symptoms → Noninvasive guided AA

Ventricular dysfunction/ischemia → Cardiac catheterization

Ischemic heart disease → Revascularization

Nonischemic cardiomyopathy → EPS not helpful, no proof yet that therapy affects survival; consider amiodarone for symptomatic arrhythmias

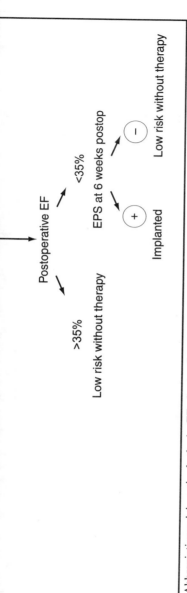

Postoperative EF

>35%   <35%

Low risk without therapy   EPS at 6 weeks postop

                            Implanted   Low risk without therapy

Abbreviations: AA, antiarrhythmic; EF, ejection fraction; EPS, electrophysiology study.

Modifed from: Curtis AB. Management of the patient at risk for sudden cardiac death. In: Mills RM, Young JB, eds. *Practical Approaches to the Treatment of Heart Failure*. Baltimore, Md: Williams and Wilkins; 1998.

10

289

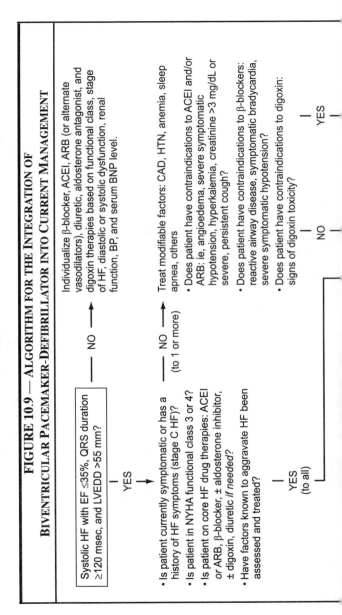

FIGURE 10.9 — ALGORITHM FOR THE INTEGRATION OF BIVENTRICULAR PACEMAKER-DEFIBRILLATOR INTO CURRENT MANAGEMENT

Systolic HF with EF ≤35%, QRS duration ≥120 msec, and LVEDD >55 mm?

— **YES** →

- Is patient currently symptomatic or has a history of HF symptoms (stage C HF)?
- Is patient in NYHA functional class 3 or 4?
- Is patient on core HF drug therapies: ACEI *or* ARB, β-blocker, ± aldosterone inhibitor, ± digoxin, diuretic *if needed*?
- Have factors known to aggravate HF been assessed and treated?

YES (to all)

— **NO** →

Individualize β-blocker, ACEI, ARB (or alternate vasodilators), diuretic, aldosterone antagonist, and digoxin therapies based on functional class, stage of HF, diastolic or systolic dysfunction, renal function, BP, and serum BNP level.

— **NO** (to 1 or more) →

Treat modifiable factors: CAD, HTN, anemia, sleep apnea, others

- Does patient have contraindications to ACEI and/or ARB: ie, angioedema, severe symptomatic hypotension, hyperkalemia, creatinine >3 mg/dL or severe, persistent cough?
- Does patient have contraindications to β-blockers: reactive airway disease, symptomatic bradycardia, severe symptomatic hypotension?
- Does patient have contraindications to digoxin: signs of digoxin toxicity?

NO — — **YES** —

STOP: Until pharmacologic and nonpharma-cologic therapies are optimized.

Do not assess for cardiac resynchronization until on core pharmacologic therapies at optimum dosing for 3 months (if β–blocker-initiated or up-titrated) or 1 month for other therapies. May begin patient education and initial screening.

NO ↑

- Is patient following low-sodium diet (2000 mg/d)?
- Is patient monitoring weight and following fluid management restrictions (as needed)?

↓ YES

- Is patient still in NYHA functional class 3 or 4 with signs/symptoms of fatigue, dyspnea, exercise intolerance, change in mentation, others?

- Is patient free of end-stage non-HF conditions with life expectancy of ≤6 months?

YES →

- Is patient post-MI for at least 1 month or post–coronary artery revascularization for at least 3 months with an EF ≤30%?

NO ↓

- Is patient at target dosing of ACEI (or alternate) and β-blocker?

- Is patient on low-dose digoxin (0.125 mg/d) and low-dose spironolactone?

- Is patient on optimum dose of loop or combina-tion diuretics/d to minimize signs/symptoms of volume overload?

YES ↙

YES ↓

- If ACEI and ARB are contraindicated, is patient on hydralazine/nitrate combination?

- If yes to β-blocker and/or digoxin contraindications, ignore β-blocker titration and/or low-dose digoxin recommendations.

YES → Consult electrophysiologist for ICD and CRT.

NO → If no other ICD indication, consult electrophysiologist for CRT.

10

Continued

Abbreviations: ACEI, angiotensin-converting enzyme inhibitor; ARB, angiotensin II receptor blocker; BNP, B-type natriuretic peptide; BP, blood pressure; CAD, coronary artery disease; CRT, cardiac resynchronization therapy; EF, ejection fraction; EPS, electrophysiology study; HF, heart failure; HTN, hypertension; ICD, implantable cardioverter defibrillator; LVEDD, left ventricular end-diastolic dimensions; MI, myocardial infarction; NYHA, New York Heart Association.

Note: EPS consultation can be performed in any setting: emergency care, inpatient, or outpatient.

TABLE 10.12 — RECENT TRIALS WITH DEVICES FOR HEART FAILURE

Trial	Criteria
COMPANION	Comparison of medical therapy, BiV-CRT, and BiV-CRT with ICD in chronic heart failure
MIRACLE ICD	RV sensor, ICD, CRT
Ventak-CHF	BiV antitachycardia pacing and defibrillation

Abbreviations: BiV, biventricular; COMPANION, Comparison of Medical Therapy, Pacing and Defibrillation in Chronic Heart Failure; CRT, cardiac resynchronization therapy; ICD, implantable cardioverter defibrillator; MIRACLE ICD, Multicenter InSync Randomized Clinic Evaluation Implantable Cardioverter Defibrillator; RV, right ventricle.

10

11 Surgical Approaches to Heart Failure

Introduction

The complexity of surgical approaches to heart failure (HF), often involving combined procedures (ie, valve repair and revascularization), and the many variables that influence surgical outcomes make objective assessment of surgical therapy substantially more difficult than assessment of new medical therapy. Nonetheless, there are many reasons to integrate surgical approaches to HF into the overall approach to HF management. Historically, surgical approaches have proven the most effective modality for relief of pressure and volume overload associated with valvular disease. Direct surgical revascularization with at least one internal mammary artery graft remains the standard of care for patients with multivessel or left main coronary disease, particularly in patients with diabetes. The surgical Maze procedure may provide restoration of sinus rhythm in many patients with atrial fibrillation (AF).

As with coronary disease, medical and surgical management are complimentary, not mutually exclusive. Just as the postbypass patient should continue with antiplatelet and lipid-lowering medical management, the HF patient who undergoes surgery should continue with neurohormonal blocking agents and comprehensive electrophysiologic care. This absolute requirement for continuing sophisticated medical care adds another layer of complexity to the evaluation of surgical outcomes for evidence-based care.

11

Table 11.1 summarizes a number of surgical approaches to structural heart disease associated with HF symptoms. The approaches include:

- Relatively standard procedures
- More highly specialized procedures generally limited to larger volume surgical centers
- Mechanical cardiac support (MCS)
- Transplantation
- Approaches under evaluation in clinical trials.

Cardiac transplantation now offers highly selected individuals the prospect of approximately 50% *10-year* survival, but the constraints placed by limited donors make transplantation epidemiologically insignificant.[100] Consequently, surgical interest in MCS has burgeoned,

---

TABLE 11.1 — SURGICAL APPROACHES TO HEART FAILURE MANAGEMENT

Accepted Evidence-Based Approaches
- Surgical revascularization for coronary disease
- Aortic valve replacement for severe aortic stenosis even with poor left ventricular function
- Orthotopic cardiac transplantation

Newer Evidence-Based Approaches
- Mitral valve repair in the setting of myopathic ventricular function
- Septal myectomy for hypertrophic cardiomyopathy
- Pulmonary thromboendarterectomy for chronic thromboembolic pulmonary hypertension

New Approaches Supported by Limited Evidence
- Postinfarction ventricular reconstruction (Dor procedure)
- Mechanical cardiac support with left ventricular assist device ("destination" therapy)

Emerging and Experimental Procedures
- Myosplint device
- Acorn device
- Total artificial heart

---

supported by the findings of the REMATCH trial.[254] The trial randomized 129 subjects with end-stage HF to receive a left ventricular assist device (LVAD) (68 subjects) or optimal medical management (61 subjects). Two-year survival was 23% in the MCS group and 8% in the medically managed group. Despite these rather discouraging long-term outcomes, even with current devices MCS clearly offers a survival advantage and has gained acceptance as "destination therapy" for some patients. Many challenges remain, including:

- Better definition of appropriate candidates
- Infection control
- Cost containment.

Nonetheless, the indications for and use of long-term MCS will almost certainly continue to expand in the coming years.

Procedures currently under active investigation include the Acorn restraining device and the Myosplint left ventricular (LV)–shape-changing device.

Hibernating Myocardium

Because revascularization of viable but noncontractile ischemic myocardium leads to improved ventricular function and improved clinical outcomes, coronary angiography and viability assessment should be considered for all patients with HF. Viability assessment can be done effectively with radionuclide techniques, including rest/redistribution thallium imaging or positron emission tomography (PET)–rubidium fluorodeoxyglucose (FDG) studies, and also with dobutamine stress echocardiography. Gadolinium magnetic resonance imaging studies are also quite helpful although difficult to perform in patients with pacers and implantable cardioverter defibrillators (ICDs), now a common situation in HF cohorts. In our view, a consistent practice of searching for coronary disease and viability is more important than the choice of assessment technique.

Figure 11.1 shows a conceptual outline of the response of hibernating myocardium to increasing coronary blood flow. Practicing physicians must appreciate potential myocardial hibernation accompanying acute and chronic ischemic syndromes and make a concerted effort to search it out. Hibernating myocardium represents viable but nonfunctional myocardium tissue that, upon restoration of normal blood flow, will be-

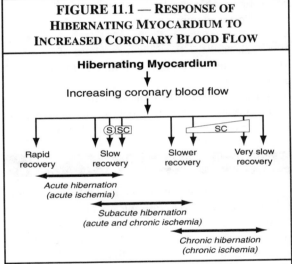

FIGURE 11.1 — RESPONSE OF HIBERNATING MYOCARDIUM TO INCREASED CORONARY BLOOD FLOW

Abbreviations: S, myocardial stunning; SC, structural changes.

The continuum of acute, subacute, and chronic hibernating myocardium, demonstrating the relationship between recovery of potentially functional myocardium that is, in fact, hibernating.

Rahimtoola SH. *Am J Cardiol.* 1995;75:16E-22E.

come functional. **Table 11.2** summarizes those conditions in which myocardial hibernation is common.

TABLE 11.2 — HEART FAILURE SUGGESTIVE OF ISCHEMIC/HIBERNATING MYOCARDIUM*

- Diabetic patients with coronary disease and heart failure
- Flash pulmonary edema patients
- Heart failure patients with multivessel coronary artery disease (CAD) but without previous documented infarction
- Multivessel occlusive CAD with extensive collateralization

* Absence of angina common.

Valve Repair or Replacement

Table 11.3 addresses mitral valve repair for HF patients with substantial left ventricular dysfunction (LVD). Until recently, LVD (LV ejection fraction [LVEF] <35%, in particular) represented a contraindication to surgical management of mitral regurgitation. However, more recent data suggests that correction of severe mitral regurgitation in patients with cardiomyopathic clinical presentations improves ventricular geometry and has a good intermediate-term outcome.[23] This radical change in thought probably represents both changes in the etiology of mitral regurgitation we are now seeing and improvement in surgical technique. Surgical approaches should be considered when mitral regurgitation is apparent with acute HF and in individuals with moderate LV systolic dysfunction and severe (3+ to 4+) mitral regurgitation with persistence of symptoms when medications have been optimized.

Aortic valve replacement in patients with critical aortic stenosis and impaired LV function can benefit virtually all who present in such fashion. In those with very severe HF, intensive and skillful preoperative HF

11

TABLE 11.3 — MITRAL VALVE REPAIR FOR HEART FAILURE WITH LEFT VENTRICULAR DYSFUNCTION

Considerations for Surgery
- Flail leaflet due to disruption of mitral apparatus
- Severe myxomatous degeneration with grade 4 regurgitant jet by Doppler
- As a combination procedure with:
  – Coronary revascularization
  – Aortic valve replacement
  – Left ventricular reconstruction surgery
- For moderate LVD (LVEF 25% to 35%) with severe MR (3+ to 4+) when afterload reduction is poorly tolerated
- In select patients with severe LVD (LVEF <20%) and severe MR (4+)

Abbreviations: LVD, left ventricular dysfunction; LVEF, left ventricular ejection fraction; MR, mitral regurgitation.

management will improve the odds of successful surgery.[147] Essentially, no EF is too low to justify withholding surgical referral in these patients.

Surgical Remodeling

Figure 11.2 depicts the focus of surgical remodeling procedures, the law of Laplace. This mathematical rule indicates that LV wall stress is related to intracavitary pressure times radius divided by LV wall thickness. As failing hearts dilate and the radius increases, wall stress increases. High wall stress stimulates detrimental remodeling processes. Surgical procedures designed to remodel LV shape by reducing chamber radius should decrease wall stress. One of the first attempts at surgical remodeling, the Batista procedure (named after Randas Batista, a Brazilian surgeon) utilized an interpapillary muscle ventricular resection in nonischemic cardiomyopathy to reshape

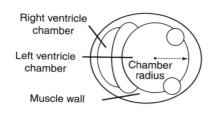

FIGURE 11.2 — FOCUS OF SURGICAL REMODELING PROCEDURES: LAW OF LAPLACE

Dilated Heart

Right ventricle chamber

Left ventricle chamber

Chamber radius

Muscle wall

$$\text{Stress} = \frac{P \leftrightarrow r}{h} = \frac{\text{Pressure} \times \text{Radius}}{\text{Wall thickness}}$$

Reduction of left ventricle (LV) radius reduces LV wall stress. If pressure or radius increases, stress increases. Surgical remodeling procedures attempt to decrease LV wall stress by reducing the radius of the ventricle.

the ventricle and reduce its radius. Despite some successes, this procedure has been abandoned because it is difficult to differentiate between those patients who will do well and those who will not.

Figure 11.3 depicts infarct-exclusion surgery. The difference between infarct-exclusion and LV volume-reduction surgery primarily rests with patient selection. The infarct-exclusion operation is done in individuals with prior anteroseptal myocardial infarction. In this procedure, the infarcted akinetic area is addressed with the heart beating while on cardiopulmonary bypass. The infarct is opened and a purse-string suture is placed at the border zone between scarred and infarcted myocardium. Tying the purse-string suture creates a net that can be closed with further sutures or a patch. Sometimes a patch is used to help properly shape the ven-

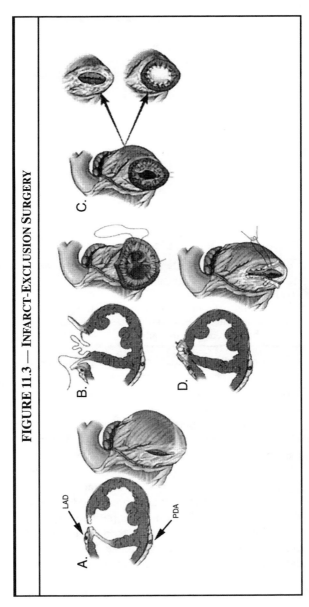

FIGURE 11.3 — INFARCT-EXCLUSION SURGERY

LAD

PDA

A.

B.

C.

D.

Abbreviations: LAD, left anterior descending [artery]; LV, left ventricle; PDA, posterior descending artery.

A: LAD infarction and akinesis produce thinning of the anterior LV free wall and septum. Previous ventricular aneurysm repairs addressed only the thinned wall, leaving the akinetic septum intact. B: With the heart beating on cardiopulmonary bypass, the infarct is opened and a purse-string suture is placed at the border zone between scarred and infarcted myocardium. C: Tying the purse-string suture creates a neck that can be closed with further sutures (above) or a patch (below). D: After reconstruction of the infarcted area, both septum and free wall are excluded from the LV cavity, reducing LV dimensions and wall stress in the remaining myocardium. This improves function in myocardium remote from the scar.

11

tricular cavity and close the gap. After reconstruction of the infarcted area, both septum and free wall are excluded from the LV cavity, reducing LV dimensions and wall stress in the remaining myocardium. This improves function in myocardium that is not ischemic and remote from the scar.

Table 11.4 summarizes the evaluation of candidates for infarct-exclusion surgery. We currently use gadolinium magnetic resonance imaging in as many patients as possible (those without pacemakers and automatic implantable cardioverter defibrillators [AICDs]) to evaluate nonviable transmural anterior apical LV scar. Otherwise, positron emission tomography (PET) scanning with fluorodeoxyglucose (FDG) is used to define ventricular scar, ischemia, and hibernation location and size. Echocardiography is used to evaluate the need for mitral and/or tricuspid valve repair.

Real-time three dimensional echocardiography at 6 to 12 months following LV reconstruction surgery (often combined with mitral valve repair and/or revascularization) has documented significant reduction in LV volumes and improvement in LV function. In these patients, recurrent mitral regurgitation is associated with increased ventricular volumes, underscoring the need for a comprehensive surgical approach to HF. In addition, many patients undergoing surgical treatment also will benefit from placement of LV epicardial leads to facilitate biventricular pacing, and most should undergo electrophysiologic evaluation at an appropriate point postsurgery.[245] Finally, if chronic AF is present, a surgical procedure for this can be added to the operative protocol (see Chapter 10, *Arrhythmia and Electrophysiologic Considerations*).

Investigational Procedures

Figure 11.4 summarizes a thought experiment that will introduce the Myosplint LV–shape-changing de-

TABLE 11.4 — EVALUATION OF CANDIDATES FOR INFARCT-EXCLUSION SURGERY

Clinical Evaluation
- Documented coronary artery disease (particularly proximal left anterior descending obstruction)
- Impaired left ventricular systolic function (LVEF <30%)
- LVESI >50 cc^2
- Anteroapical akinesia and/or dyskinesia documented
- Absence of major comorbidity:
  - Carotid artery occlusions
  - Abdominal aortic disease
  - Renal dysfunction
  - Severe pulmonary disease

Laboratory Evaluation
- Cardiac MRI with gadolinium or PET scan with FDG to confirm nonviable transmural anteroapical left ventricular scar and adequate functional myocardium for reconstruction
- Echocardiography to evaluate need for mitral and/or tricuspid repair
- Coronary angiography to assess suitability for revascularization of viable segments

Postoperative Evaluation and Management
- Electrophysiologic testing for AICD consideration
- Consider BiV-CRT LV pacer hookup
- ACEI, β-blockers, antiplatelet therapy, statins

11

Abbreviations: ACE, angiotensin-converting enzyme inhibitors; AICD, automatic implantable cardioverter defibrillator; BiV, biventricular; CRT, cardiac resynchronization therapy; FDG, fluorodeoxyglucose; LV, left ventricular; LVEF, left ventricular ejection fraction; LVESI, left ventricular end-systolic index; MRI, magnetic resonance imaging; PET, positron emission tomography.

vice. One can imagine two individuals holding a sail against which a breeze is blowing. LV wall stress would be analogous to the tension at the end (sheets) of the sail with which the two individuals must grapple. As the sail moves forward into the forestay, the stress (tension) is significantly diminished. If one translates this concept into a large globular left ventricle, one can see that by passing a splint across the ventricle, shape change is likely to ensue with diminution of wall stress. **Figure 11**.5 is a graphic representation of how these splinting devices can be placed in the left ventricle to change a large globular-shaped ventricle into a bilobe. Experimental studies and early clinical observations suggest that this approach may be advantageous in some HF patients. There is also the possibility that mitral regurgitation can be decreased based on where the splints are placed.

The Acorn cardiac support device is an alternative shape-changing strategy. This device is a fabric mesh that encompasses the heart and is designed to prevent progressive cardiac dilation. As with the Myosplint concept, this device may improve cardiac function by helping to maintain a more normal LV shape.

Cardiac Transplantation

Despite the inherent drama of the procedure, cardiac transplantation per se has made no significant impact on HF as a public health problem. However, the ripple effects of transplantation have dramatically benefited a vast population. Cardiac transplant programs have concentrated medical and surgical specialists in HF management in academic referral centers, spurring the rapid development of new surgical approaches to HF and greatly facilitating recruitment for clinical trials in medical management. Limited donor organ availability and the complications of chronic immunosuppression continue to hamper transplantation. Pa-

FIGURE 11.4 — ANALOGY FOR CONCEPT OF MYOSPLINT

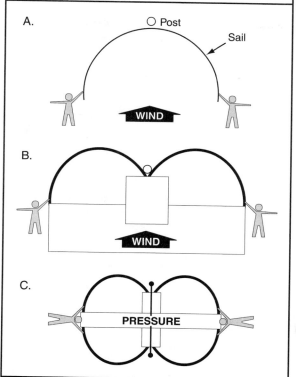

A: Stress is felt by two sailors attempting to control a large sail (ventricle) filled with wind (volume). *B:* Running the sail into the forestay makes control easier by reducing wall stress. *C:* Splinted chamber has reduced stress, like the sail in panel B.

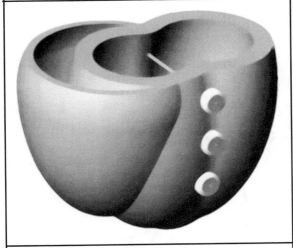

Stress reduction through ventricular shape change.

tients should be referred to a transplant center for evaluation if significant functional limitation (New York Heart Association [NYHA] III-IV) persists despite optimal management.

Given the limited donor supply and the multiple contraindications to transplantation, patients who may be candidates should be referred for specialized evaluation and management, not for "a heart transplant because there's nothing else that can be done." In the evaluation process, all possible alternatives to transplantation should be considered, including:

- Revascularization for significant reversible ischemia
- Valve replacement for critical aortic valve disease
- Valve repair or replacement for severe mitral regurgitation

- Ventricular remodeling procedures
- Biventricular pacing/ICD strategies.

Table 11.5 details the contraindications to transplantation. Evaluations for transplantation should be designed to determine the:
- Severity of the patient's illness
- Degree of HF therapeutic optimization
- Presence of comorbidities that might adversely affect clinical outcomes after cardiac transplantation.

TABLE 11.5 — CARDIAC TRANSPLANTATION: INDICATIONS AND EVALUATION

Transplantation Considerations
- Significant functional limitation (NYHA-FC III/IV)
- Refractory angina or refractory life-threatening arrhythmia that cannot be effectively treated
- Following exclusion of all surgical alternatives to transplantation such as:
  - Revascularization for significant reversible ischemia
  - Valve replacement for critical aortic valve disease
  - Valve repair or replacement for severe mitral regurgitation
  - Ventricular remodeling procedures
  - Biventricular pacing/ICD strategies

Contraindications to Transplantation
- Noncardiac systemic disease significantly reducing life expectancy or producing major function limitation
- Chronic/active infection
- Unresolved malignancy
- Patients with current alcohol, tobacco, illicit drug use, or antisocial behavior
- Demonstrated noncompliance with medical treatment
- Severe obesity (>150% ideal body weight) or BMI >35

Relative Contraindications to Transplantation
- Pulmonary vascular resistance of >5 Wood units after drug testing
- FEV_1 <1 L or 50% of predicted
- Serum creatinine >3 or creatinine clearance <30 cc/min
- Age >70 years
- Diabetes with advanced systemic complications (neuropathy or vasculopathy)

Evaluations
- Metabolic exercise testing (VO_{2max} determination)
- Complete hemodynamic evaluation and screening for reversibility of pulmonary hypertension
- Thorough metabolic evaluations
- Search for significant comorbidities

Continued

Specific Recommendations
- Definite indications:
  - VO_{2max} <10 mL/kg/min or <55% predicted
  - NYHA-FC IV despite optimal therapy and other options being unsuitable
  - Recurrent hospitalizations for decompensated heart failure
  - Refractory ischemia with inoperable coronary artery disease and severe left ventricular ejection fraction
  - Recurrent refractory symptomatic ventricular arrhythmias that cannot be controlled

Abbreviations: BMI, body mass index; FEV_1, forced expiratory volume in one second; ICD, implantable cardioverter defibrillator; NYHA-FC, New York Heart Association functional class; VO_{2max}, peak oxygen consumption.

12 Guidelines for Heart Failure Management

Introduction

The widespread introduction of diagnostic and management guidelines into the clinical literature began in the late 1980s and early 1990s. The guidelines movement represents an effort to synthesize available evidence about the management of a clinical problem into a set of recommendations for best practice. Well-written guidelines are systematically derived statements that evaluate the quality of data available to inform clinical decision-making. Most guidelines reflect the consensus of a panel of acknowledged experts in the field. In general, a well-constructed practice guideline:

- Specifies the qualifications of the individuals involved in guideline development
- Defines the strategy used to identify primary evidence
- Provides a clear grading of recommendations.

Table 12.1 points out a number of problems with clinical practice guidelines. Guidelines cannot address all clinical situations. Often consensus cannot be achieved because evidence is not always available regarding certain therapeutic strategies.[225] Furthermore, guidelines are slow to incorporate new knowledge and therapies. It is also difficult to educate clinicians regarding guidelines, and some perceive them as unduly regulatory and intrusive.

Currently available data suggest that strategies designed to improve physician compliance with guidelines largely fail to do so. Neither active reminders

TABLE 12.1 — CLINICAL PRACTICE GUIDELINES

Importance/Relevance
- Provide response to significant clinical challenge
- Recognize consensus regarding screening, diagnosis, and treatments of significant diseases
- Primarily evidence based
- Educational tools
- Establish quality practice standards

Problems
- Guidelines cannot address all clinical situations
- Often cannot identify consensus
- Evidence not always available
- Changing guidelines is ponderous process
- Slow to incorporate new knowledge/therapies
- Difficult to educate clinicians
- Guidelines perceived as regulatory and an unduly intrusive nuisance

from electronic systems nor passive distribution of printed guidelines impacted heart failure (HF) management in two recent studies.[288,293] However, accreditation organizations and third-party payers have begun to incorporate adherence to guidelines into their criteria for assessing medical quality. This growing focus on evidence-based quality indicators will almost certainly impact physician behaviors.

Available Guidelines

Table 12.2 lists clinical HF treatment guidelines beginning with the US Department of Health and Human Services Agency for Health Care Policy and Research (AHCPR) guidelines of 1994.[24-26,87,152] The list includes only English-language publications. Several European medical organizations have also published excellent guidelines.

The most common themes of the HF guidelines collectively are summarized in **Table 12.3**. All guidelines suggest aggressive identification and treatment of active ischemia in patients with HF. The guidelines are unanimous in recommending angiotensin-converting enzyme inhibitors (ACEIs) in all patients who can tolerate these drugs when systolic left ventricular dysfunction (LVD) (generally of any degree) is present. More recent guidelines address the use of β-blockers in stable patients with mild-to-moderate symptoms and no significant congestion. All guidelines suggest avoiding agents with incomplete benefit-risk profiles and remind clinicians about diagnosing and addressing underlying and precipitating disorders. Furthermore, most guidelines emphasize the importance of prescribing non-pharmacologic therapy such as exercise and salt and fluid restriction while addressing patient education.

Unfortunately, HF guidelines published to date have not addressed several important areas. HF with preserved LV systolic function, management of advanced HF, and management of acutely decompensated HF have not been specifically addressed. **Table 12.4** lists some useful special situation guidelines that have been recently published. Final consensus has not yet been reached about best use of angiotensin receptor blockers, biventricular pacers, implantable cardiac defibrillators, and surgical or electrophysiologic manipulations.

Guidelines have defined areas of consensus and specific issues where no consensus exists in HF management. Generating quality guidelines demands time, resources, and the involvement of acknowledged experts. We support the efforts of the major professional organizations in cardiovascular medicine to continually update the standards of best-care practice. Their efforts give practicing physicians who avail themselves of the information invaluable support in their care of patients with complex situations in HF.

12

TABLE 12.2 — CLINICAL HEART FAILURE TREATMENT GUIDELINES

Research Group for Heart Failure Guidelines	Year Published	Reference
US Department of Health and Human Services, Agency for Health Care Policy and Research (AHCPR)	1994	AHCPR Publication No. 94-0612: June 1994.
American College of Cardiology/American Heart Association (ACC/AHA) Task Force Practice Guidelines (Committee on Evaluation and Management of Heart Failure)	1995	*Circulation.* 1995;92:2764-2784.
World Health Organization (WHO) Heart Failure Guidelines	1996	*J Card Fail.* 1996;2:153-155.
Task Force of the Working Group on Heart Failure of the European Society of Cardiology	1997	*Eur Heart J.* 1997;18:736-753.
Advisory Council to Improve Outcomes Nationwide (ACTION) Heart Failure Guidelines	1999	*Am J Cardiol.* 1999;83(2A):1A-38A.
Heart Failure Society of America (HFSA) Practice Guidelines	1999	*J Card Fail.* 1999;5:357-382.
National Heart, Lung, and Blood Institute (NHLBI) and Office of Rare Diseases (National Institutes of Health [NIH])	2000	*JAMA.* 2000;283:1183-1188.
Working Group on Cardiac Rehabilitation and Exercise Physiology and Working Group on Heart Failure of the European Society of Cardiology (exercise testing)	2001	*Eur Heart J.* 2001;22:37-45.

Working Group on Cardiac Rehabilitation and Exercise Physiology and Working Group on Heart Failure of the European Society of Cardiology (exercise training)	2001	*Eur Heart J.* 2001;22:125-135.
ACC/AHA Task Force Practice Guidelines (Committee to revise the 1995 Guidelines for the Evaluation and Management of Heart Failure)	2001	*Circulation.* 2001;104:2996-3007.
Task Force for the Diagnosis and Treatment of Chronic Heart Failure, European Society of Cardiology	2001	*Eur Heart J.* 2001;22:1527-1560.
Task Force on Sudden Cardiac Death of the European Society of Cardiology	2001	*Eur Heart J.* 2001;22:1374-1450.
Canadian Cardiovascular Society Consensus Guideline (Update for the Management and Prevention of Heart Failure)	2001	*Can J Cardiol.* 2001;17(Suppl E):5E-25E.
European Society of Cardiology (Update of the Guidelines on Sudden Cardiac Death)	2003	*Eur Heart J.* 2003;24:13-15.
AHA Committee on Exercise, Rehabilitation, and Prevention	2003	*Circulation.* 2003;107:1210-1225.
International Society for Heart and Lung Transplantation	2003	*J Heart Lung Transplant.* 2003;22:365-369.
Canadian Cardiovascular Society Consensus Guideline (Update for the Diagnosis and Management of Heart Failure)	2003	*Can J Cardiol.* 2003;19:347-356.

12

TABLE 12.3 — MOST COMMON THEMES OF HEART FAILURE GUIDELINES

- Identify and aggressively treat ischemia in patients with heart failure (revascularization)
- Use ACEIs in all patients with left ventricular systolic dysfunction who tolerate them
- Use ARBs in ACEI–intolerant patients
- Use β-blockers in stable patients with mild-to-moderate symptoms and no significant congestion
- Low-dose β-blocker therapy may be initiated in NYHA Class III-IV patients
- Avoid agents with incomplete benefit/risk profiles
- Diagnose and address underlying/precipitating disorders
- Prescribe nonpharmacologic therapies:
  - Exercise
  - Salt/fluid restriction
- Educate patient, family, and caregivers

Abbreviations: ACEI, angiotensin-converting enzyme inhibitor; ARB, angiotensin receptor blocker; NYHA, New York Heart Association.

TABLE 12.4 — GUIDELINES FOR SPECIAL SITUATIONS IN HEART FAILURE			
Research Group	Special Condition With Heart Failure	Year Published	Reference
National Heart, Lung, and Blood Institute (NHLBI) and Office of Rare Diseases (National Institutes of Health [NIH])	Peripartum cardiomyopathy	2000	*JAMA.* 2000;283:1183-1188.
Council on the Kidney in Cardiovascular Disease and the Council for High Blood Pressure Research for the American Heart Association (AHA)	Renal considerations in angiotensin-converting enzyme inhibition therapy	2001	*Circulation.* 2001;104:1985-1991.
American College of Cardiology/American Heart Association/North American Society for Pacing and Electrophysiology (ACC/AHA/NASPE)	Implantation of pace-makers and antiar-rhythmia devices	2002	*Circulation.* 2002;106:2145-2161.
American Academy of Family Physicians/ American College of Physicians (AAFP/ACP)	Newly detected atrial fibrillation	2003	*Ann Intern Med.* 2003;139:1009-1017.

12

Continued

Research Group	Special Condition With Heart Failure	Year Published	Reference
American College of Cardiology/American Heart Association/American Society for Nuclear Cardiology (ACC/AHA/ASNC)	Clinical use of cardiac radionuclide imaging	2003	*J Am Coll Cardiol.* 2003;42:1318-1333.
American Heart Association/American Diabetes Association (AHA/ADA)	Thiazolidinedione use, fluid retention, and congestive heart failure	2003	*Circulation.* 2003;108:2941-2948.

13   List of Trial Acronyms

ACCLAIM: Advanced Chronic Heart Failure Clinical Assessment of Immune Modulation[292]

ADOPT-A: Atrial Dynamic Overdrive Pacing Trial[54]

AFT: Atrial Fibrillation Therapy [trial][135]

AIRE: Acute Infarction Ramipril Efficacy[6]

AIREX: Acute Infarction Ramipril Efficacy Extension [study][118]

ALLHAT: Antihypertensive and Lipid-Lowering Treatment to Prevent Heart Attack Trial[10,159]

AMIOVERT: Amiodarone vs ICD in IDC Mortality Trial[283]

APRES: Angiotensin-Converting Enzyme Inhibition Post Revascularization Study[148]

ASPECT: Atrial Septal Pacing Efficacy Clinical Trial[220]

AT500: Pace-termination and pacing for prevention of atrial tachyarrhythmias; AT500 Verification Study[136]

ATLAS: Assessment of Treatment With Lisinopril and Survival[34,218,259,296]

ATTEST: Atrial Therapy Efficacy and Safety Trial[163]

AVID: Antiarrhythmics vs Implantable Defibrillators [trial][14,92,201]

BASIS: Basal Antiarrhythmic Study of Infarct Survival[43]

BEST: β-Blocker Evaluation of Survival Trial[31]

BNP: Breathing Not Properly [study][186]

CABG Patch: Coronary Artery Bypass Graft Patch [trial][34,78]

CAMIAT: Canadian Amiodarone Myocardial Infarction Arrhythmia Trial[47,48]

CAPPP: Captopril Prevention Project[122]

CAPRICORN: Carvedilol Post-Infarction Survival Control in Left Ventricular Dysfunction[50]

CARE-HF: Cardiac Resynchronization in Heart Failure[323]

EPHESUS: Eplerenone Neurohormonal Efficacy and Survival Study[233,235]

ESCAPE: Evaluation Study of Congestive Heart Failure and Pulmonary Artery Catheterization Effectiveness[260]

FACET: Flosequinan ACE Inhibitor Trial[184]

FIRST: Flolan International Randomized Survival Trial[49]

GESICA: Grupo de Estudio de la Sobrevida en la Insuficiencia Cardiaca en Argentina[86]

Growth Hormone: Preliminary Study of Growth Hormone in the Treatment of Dilated Cardiomyopathy[94,171]

HOPE: Heart Outcomes Prevention Evaluation[124-127,172,196,274]

HY-C: Hydralazine vs Captopril: Effect on Mortality in Patients With Advanced Heart Failure[98]

IMAC: Intervention in Myocarditis and Acute Cardiomyopathy With IV Immunoglobulin[190]

IMPRESS: Inhibition of Metalloprotease by BMS-186716 in a Randomized Exercise and Symptoms Study[255]

LIDO: Levosimendan Infusion vs Dobutamine [in low output heart failure][221]

MACH-I: Mortality Assessment in Congestive Heart Failure I[166]

MADIT: Multicenter Automatic Defibrillator Implantation Trial[198,199]

MDC: Metoprolol in Dilated Cardiomyopathy[301]

MERIT-HF: Metoprolol CR/XL Randomized Intervention Trial in Heart Failure[129,191]

MHFT: Munich Mild Heart Failure Trial[149]

MEXIS: Metoprolol and Xamoterol in Ischemic Syndromes[226]

MICRO-HOPE: Microalbuminuria, Cardiovascular, and Renal Outcomes–HOPE [substudy][125]

MIRACLE: Multicenter InSync Randomization Clinical Evaluation [North America][1,2,3,75,281]

MIRACLE ICD: Multicenter InSync Randomization Clinical Evaluation Implantable Cardioverter Defibrillator[193]

MOCHA: Multicenter Oral Carvedilol Heart Failure Assessment[39]

MOXCON: Moxonidine in Congestive Heart Failure[140,285]

13

MUSTIC: Multisite Stimulation Cardiomyopathy [trial][55,162,169]

MUSTT: Multicenter Unsustained Tachycardia Trial[44,45,201]

Myocarditis Treatment Trial: A Clinical Trial of Immunosuppressive Therapy for Myocarditis[183]

OPTIME-CHF: Outcomes of a Prospective Trial of Intravenous Milrinone for Exacerbation of Chronic Heart Failure[105]

OVERTURE: Omapatrilat vs Enalapril Randomized Trial of Utility in Reducing Events[211]

PATH-CHF: Pacing Therapies for Congestive Heart Failure[18-20]

PIAF: Pharmacological Intervention in Atrial Fibrillation[134]

PICO: Pimobendan in Congestive Heart Failure[230]

PIPAF: Pacing in Prevention of Atrial Fibrillation[258]

PRAISE: Prospective Randomized Amlodipine Survival Evaluation[104,217]

PRECISE/MOCHA: Prospective Randomized Evaluation of Carvedilol on Symptoms and Exercise/Multicenter Oral Carvedilol Heart Failure Assessment[214]

PRIME: Second Prospective Randomized Study of Ibopamine on Mortality and Efficacy[121,178]

PROFILE: Prospective Randomized Flosequinan Longevity Evaluation[195,242]

PROMISE: Prospective Randomized Milrinone Survival Evaluation[207,212]

PROVED: Prospective Randomized Study of Ventricular Failure and the Efficacy of Digoxin[297,317]

RADIANCE: Randomized Assessment of Digoxin and Inhibitors of Angiotensin-Converting Enzyme[215]

RALES: Randomized Aldactone Evaluation Study[29,236,251,304,322]

REFLECT: Randomized Evaluation of Flosequinan on Exercise Tolerance[216]

REMATCH: Randomized Evaluation of Mechanical Assistance Therapy as an Alternative in Congestive Heart Failure[254]

RENAISSANCE: Randomized Etanercept North American Strategy to Study Antagonism of Cytokines[89]

RESOLVD: Randomized Evaluation of Strategies for Left Ventricular Dysfunction[111,188,248,294]

RESOLVD (Metoprolol Study): Randomized Evaluation of Strategies for Left Ventricular Dysfunction–β-Blocker[111,188,248,294]

RITZ: Randomized Intravenous Tezosentan[291]

SAVE: Survival and Ventricular Enlargement[227]

SCD-HeFT: Sudden Cardiac Death–Heart Failure Trial[27,324]

SHOCK: Should We Emergently Revascularize Occluded Coronaries for Cardiogenic Shock[131-133]

SMILE: Survival of Myocardial Infarction: Long-Term Evaluation[11]

SOLVD: Studies of Left Ventricular Dysfunction [treatment and prevention trials][37,91,155,190,276-278]

SPICE-Registry: Study of Patients Intolerant of Converting Enzyme Inhibitors [clinical registry][28,109,259]

SPICE-Trial: Study of Patients Intolerant of Converting Enzyme Inhibitors [clinical trial][28,109,259]

STRETCH: Symptom, Tolerability, Response to Exercise Trial of Candesartan Cilexetil in Heart Failure[252]

SUPPORT: Study to Understand Prognoses and Preferences for Outcomes and Risks of Treatment[137]

SWORD: Survival With Oral *d*-Sotalol[302]

TRACE: Trandolapril Cardiac Evaluation[151,289]

VaL-HeFT: Valsartan Heart Failure Trial[67,68]

VALIANT: Valsartan in Acute Myocardial Infarction Trial[298]

VEST: Vesnarinone Evaluation of Survival Trial[65,95,96]

V-HeFT: Vasodilator-Heart Failure Trial I[15,35,64,66,69]

VMAC: Vasodilation in the Management of Acute Congestive Heart Failure[319]

WATCH: Warfarin Anticoagulation Trial in CHF[138,139]

Xamoterol: Xamoterol in Severe Heart Failure[309]

For a more complete list of clinical trials relevant to cardiovascular disease in general, see:

Kloner RA, Birnbaum Y, Chi J. *Cardiovascular Trials Review*. 8th ed. Greenwich, Conn: LeJacq Communications; 2003.

14 References

1. Abraham W, for the MIRACLE Investigators. *Late Breaking Clinical Trials.* American College of Cardiology. Orlando, Fla. March, 2001.

2. Abraham WT, Fisher W, Smith A, et al. Long-term improvement in functional status, quality of life and exercise capacity with cardiac resynchronization therapy: the MIRACLE trial experience. *J Am Coll Cardiol.* 2002;39: 159A. Abstract.

3. Abraham WT, Fisher WG, Smith AL, et al. Cardiac resynchronization in chronic heart failure. *N Engl J Med.* 2002;346:1845-1853.

4. Abraham WT, Lowes BD, Ferguson DA, et al. Systemic hemodynamic, neurohormonal, and renal effects of a steady-state infusion of human brain natriuretic peptide in patients with hemodynamically decompensated heart failure. *J Card Fail.* 1998;4:37-44.

5. Abrams J. Beneficial actions of nitrates in cardiovascular disease. *Am J Cardiol.* 1996;77:31c-37c.

6. Acute Infarction Ramipril Efficacy (AIRE) Study Investigators. Effect of ramipril on mortality and morbidity of survivors of acute myocardial infarction with clinical evidence of heart failure. *Lancet.* 1993;342:821-828.

7. Akosah KO, Schaper AM, Havlik P, et al. Improving care for patients with chronic heart failure in the community: the importance of a disease management program. *Chest.* 2002;122:906-912.

8. Alderman EL, Fisher LD, Litwin P, et al. Results of coronary artery surgery in patients with poor left ventricular function (CASS). *Circulation.* 1983;68:785-795.

9. Al-Khadra AS, Salem DN, Rand WM, Udelson JE, Smith JJ, Konstam MA. Warfarin anticoagulation and survival: a cohort analysis from the Studies of Left Ventricular Dysfunction. *J Am Coll Cardiol.* 1998;31:749-753.

10. ALLHAT Collaborative Research Group. Major cardiovascular events in hypertensive patients randomized to doxazosin vs. chlorthalidone: the antihypertensive and lipid-lowering treatment to prevent heart attack trial (ALLHAT). *JAMA.* 2000;283:1967-1975.

11. Ambrosioni E, Borghi C, Magnani B. The effect of the angiotensin-converting-enzyme inhibitor zofenopril on mortality and morbidity after anterior myocardial infarction. The Survival of Myocardial Infarction Long-Term Evaluation (SMILE) Study Investigators. *N Engl J Med.* 1995;332:80-85.

12. Amiodarone Trials Meta-Analysis Investigators. Effect of prophylactic amiodarone on mortality after acute myocardial infarction and in congestive heart failure: meta-analysis of individual data from 6500 patients in randomised trials. *Lancet.* 1997;350:1417-1424.

13. Anand IS, Fisher LD, Chiang YT, et al. Changes in brain natriuretic peptide and norepinephrine over time and mortality and morbidity in the Valsartan Heart Failure Trial (Val-HeFT). *Circulation.* 2003;107:1278-1283.

14. The Antiarrhythmics Versus Implantable Defibrillators (AVID) Investigators. A comparison of antiarrhythmic- drug therapy with implantable defibrillators in patients resuscitated from near-fatal ventricular arrhythmias. *N Engl J Med.* 1997;337:1576-1583.

15. Armstrong PW, Moe GW. Medical advances in the treatment of congestive heart failure. *Circulation.* 1993;88:2941-2952.

16. Arnold JMO. Felodipine in addition to enalapril did not improve clinical status, functional capacity or ventricular function in patients with CHF. *Evidence-Based Cardiovasc Med.* March, 1998:18.

17. Assessment of Treatment With Lisinopril (ATLAS) Study Group. *Clinical Trial Operations Manual.* 1990.

18. Auricchio A, Stellbrink C, Block M, et al. Effect of pacing chamber and atrioventricular delay on acute systolic function of paced patients with congestive heart failure. The Pacing Therapies for Congestive Heart Failure Study Group. The Guidant Congestive Heart Failure Research Group. *Circulation.* 1999;99:2993-3001.

19. Auricchio A, Stellbrink C, Sack S, et al. Long-term clinical effect of hemodynamically optimized cardiac resynchronization therapy in patients with heart failure and ventricular conduction delay. *J Am Coll Cardiol.* 2002;39:2026-2033.

20. Auricchio A, Stellbrink C, Sack S, et al. The Pacing Therapies for Congestive Heart Failure (PATH-CHF) study: rationale, design, and end-points of a prospective randomized multicenter study. *Am J Cardiol.* 1999;83:130D-135D.

21. Australia-New Zealand Heart Failure Research Collaborative Group. Effects of carvedilol, a vasodilator-beta-blocker, in patients with congestive heart failure due to ischemic heart disease. *Circulation.* 1995;92:212-218.

14

22. Australia/New Zealand Heart Failure Research Collaborative Group. Randomised, placebo-controlled trial of carvedilol in patients with congestive heart failure due to ischaemic heart disease. *Lancet.* 1997;349:375-380.

23. Badhwar V, Bolling SF. Mitral valve surgery in the patient with left ventricular dysfunction. *Semin Thorac Cardiovasc Surg.* 2002;14:133-136.

24. Baker DW, Jones R, Hodges J, Massie BM, Konstam MA, Rose EA. Management of heart failure. III. The role of revascularization in the treatment of patients with moderate or severe left ventricular systolic dysfunction. *JAMA.* 1994;272:1528-1534.

25. Baker DW, Konstam MA, Bottorff M, Pitt B. Management of heart failure. I. Pharmacologic treatment. *JAMA.* 1994;272:1361-1366.

26. Baker DW, Wright RF. Management of heart failure. IV. Anticoagulation for patients with heart failure due to left ventricular systolic dysfunction. *JAMA.* 1994;272:1614-1618.

27. Bardy GH. The Sudden Cardiac Death-Heart Failure Trial (SCD-HeFT). In: Woosley RL, Singh SN, eds. *Arrhythmia Treatment and Therapy: Evaluation of Clinical Trial Evidence.* Boston: Marcel Dekker; 2000.

28. Bart BA, Ertl G, Held P, et al. Contemporary management of patients with left ventricular systolic dysfunction. Results from the Study of Patients Intolerant of Converting Enzyme Inhibitors (SPICE) Registry. *Eur Heart J.* 1999;20:1182-1190.

29. Bauersachs J, Fraccarollo D, Ertl G, Gretz N, Wehling M, Christ M. Striking increase of natriuresis by low-dose spironolactone in congestive heart failure only in combination with ACE inhibition: mechanistic evidence to support RALES. *Circulation.* 2000;102:2325-2328.

30. Baughman KL. B-type natriuretic peptide – a window to the heart. *N Engl J Med.* 2002;347:158-159.

31. The Beta-Blocker Evaluation of Survival Trial Investigators. A trial of the beta-blocker bucindolol in patients with advanced chronic heart failure. *N Engl J Med.* 2001;344:1659-1667.

32. Beta-blocker Heart Attack Trial Research Group. A randomized trial of propranolol in patients with acute myocardial infarction. I. Mortality results. *JAMA* 1982;247:1707-1714.

33. Bigger JT Jr, Fleiss JL, Rolnitzky LM, Merab JP, Ferrick KJ. Effect of digitalis treatment on survival after acute myocardial infarction. *Am J Cardiol.* 1985;55:623-630.

34. Bigger JT Jr, for the Coronary Artery Bypass Graft (CABG) Patch Trial Investigators. Prophylactic use of implanted cardiac defibrillators in patients at high risk for ventricular arrhythmias after coronary-artery bypass graft surgery. *N Engl J Med.* 1997;337:1569-1575.

35. Boden WE, Ziesche S, Carson PE, Conrad CH, Syat D, Cohn JN. Rationale and design of the third vasodilator-heart failure trial (V-HeFT III): felodipine as adjunctive therapy to enalapril and loop diuretics with or without digoxin in chronic congestive heart failure. V-HeFT III investigators. *Am J Cardiol.* 1996;77:1078-1082.

36. Bonn D. Antihypertensive drugs can affect intellectual function. *Lancet.* 1997;350:1753.

37. Bourassa MG, Gurne O, Bangdiwala SI, et al. Natural history and patterns of current practice in heart failure. The Studies of Left Ventricular Dysfunction (SOLVD) Investigators. *J Am Coll Cardiol.* 1993;22(suppl A):14A-19A.

38. Bristow MR, Feldman AM, Saxon LA. Heart failure management using implantable devices for ventricular resynchronization: Comparison of Medical Therapy, Pacing, and Defibrillation in Chronic Heart Failure (COMPANION) trial. COMPANION Steering Committee and COMPANION Clinical Investigators. *J Card Fail.* 2000;6:276-285.

39. Bristow MR, Gilbert EM, Abraham WT, et al. Carvedilol produces dose-related improvements in left ventricular function and survival in subjects with chronic heart failure. MOCHA Investigators. *Circulation.* 1996;94:2807-2816.

40. Brophy JM, Joseph L, Rouleau JL. Beta-blockers in congestive heart failure. A Bayesian meta-analysis. *Ann Intern Med.* 2001;134:550-560.

41. Burch GE, Walsh JJ, Black WC. Value of prolonged bed rest in management of cardiomegaly. *JAMA* 1963;183:81-87.

42. Burger AJ, Horton DP, LeJemtel T, et al. Effect of nesiritide (B-type natriuretic pepetide) and dobutamine on ventricular arrythmias in the treatment of patients with acutely decompensated congestive heart failure: the PRECEDENT study. *Am Heart J.* 2002;144:1102-1108.

43. Burkart F, Pfisterer M, Kiowski W, Follath F, Burckhardt D. Effect of antiarrhythmic therapy on mortality in survivors of myocardial infarction with asymptomatic complex ventricular arrhythmias: Basel Antiarrhythmic Study of Infarct Survival (BASIS). *J Am Coll Cardiol.* 1990;16:1711-1718.

44. Buxton AE, Lee KL, Di Carlo L, et al. Electrophysiologic testing to identify patients with coronary artery disease who are at risk for sudden death. Multicenter Unsustained Tachycardia Trial Investigators. *N Engl J Med.* 2000;342:1937-1945.

45. Buxton AE, Lee KL, Fisher JD, et al. A randomized study of the prevention of sudden death in patients with coronary artery disease: Multicenter Unsustained Tachycardia Trial Investigators. *N Engl J Med.* 1999;341:1882-1890.

14

46. Byington R, Goldstein S. Association of digitalis therapy with mortality in survivors of acute myocardial infarction: observations in the Beta-Blocker Heart Attack Trial. *J Am Coll Cardiol.* 1985;6:976-982.

47. Cairns JA, Connolly SJ, Roberts R, Gent M. Canadian Amiodarone Myocardial Infarction Arrhythmia Trial (CAMIAT): rationale and protocol. CAMIAT Investigators. *Am J Cardiol.* 1993;72:87F-94F.

48. Cairns JA, Connolly SJ, Roberts R, Gent M. Randomised trial of outcome after myocardial infarction in patients with frequent or repetitive ventricular premature depolarisations: CAMIAT. Canadian Amiodarone Myocardial Infarction Arrhythmia Trial Investigators. *Lancet.* 1997;349:675-682.

49. Califf RM, Adams KF, McKenna WJ, et al. A randomized controlled trial of epoprostenol therapy for severe congestive heart failure: The Flolan International Randomized Survival Trial (FIRST). *Am Heart J.* 1997;134:44-54.

50. The CAPRICORN Investigators. The effect of carvedilol on outcome after myocardial infarction in patients with left ventricular dysfunction. The CAPRICORN randomised trial. *Lancet.* 2001;357:1385-1370.

51. The Cardiac Arrhythmia Pilot Study (CAPS) Investigators. Effects of encainide, flecainide, imipramine and moricizine on ventricular arrhythmias during the year after acute myocardial infarction: the CAPS. *Am J Cardiol.* 1988;61:501-509.

52. The Cardiac Arrhythmia Suppression Trial II Investigators. Effect of the antiarrhythmic agent moricizine on survival after myocardial infarction. *N Engl J Med.* 1992;327:227-333.

53. The Cardiac Arrhythmia Suppression Trial (CAST) Investigators. Preliminary report: effect of encainide and flecainide on mortality in a randomized trial of arrhythmia suppression after myocardial infarction. *N Engl J Med.* 1989;321:406-412.

54. Carlson MD, Gold MR, Ip J, et al. Dynamic atrial overdrive pacing decreases symptomatic atrial arrhythmia burden in patients with sinus node dysfunction. *Circulation.* 2001;104(suppl):II-383. Abstract 1825.

55. Cazeau S, Leclercq C, Lavergne T, et al. Effects of multisite biventricular pacing in patients with heart failure and intraventricular conduction delay. *N Engl J Med.* 2001;344:873-880.

56. Ceremuzynski L, Kleczar E, Krzeminska-Pakula M, et al. Effect of amiodarone on mortality after myocardial infarction: a double-blind, placebo-controlled pilot study. *J Am Coll Cardiol.* 1992;20:1056-1062.

57. Chatterjee K. Heart failure therapy in evolution. *Circulation* 1996;94:2689-2693. Editorial.

58. Chen MS, Marrouche N, et al. Pulmonary vein isolation for treatment of atrial fibrillation in patients with impaired systolic function. Presented at The Annual Meeting of the American College of Cardiology; March 2002; Atlanta, Ga. Abstract.

59. Chen SA, Hsieh MH, Tai CT, et al. Initiation of atrial fibrillation by ectopic beats originating from the pulmonary veins: electrophysiological characteristics, pharmacological responses, and effects of radiofrequency ablation. *Circulation.* 1999;100:1879-1886.

60. Cheng TO. Acronyms of clinical trials in cardiology—1996. *J Am Coll Cardiol.* 1996;27:1293-1305.

61. CIBIS Investigators and Committees. A randomized trial of beta-blockade in heart failure. The Cardiac Insufficiency Bisoprolol Study (CIBIS). *Circulation.* 1994;90: 1765-1773.

62. CIBIS-II Investigators and Committees. The Cardiac Insufficiency Bisoprolol Study II (CIBIS-II): a randomised trial. *Lancet.* 1999;353:9-13.

63. Cohn JN. The management of chronic heart failure. *N Engl J Med.* 1996;335:490-498.

64. Cohn JN, Archibald DG, Ziesche S, et al. Effect of vasodilator therapy on mortality in chronic congestive heart failure. Results of a Veterans Administration Cooperative Study. *N Engl J Med.* 1986;314:1547-1552.

65. Cohn JN, Goldstein SO, Greenberg BH, et al. A dose-dependent increase in mortality with vesnarinone among patients with severe heart failure. Vesnarinone Trial Investigators. *N Engl J Med.* 1998;339:1810-1816.

66. Cohn JN, Johnson G, Ziesche S, et al. A comparison of enalapril with hydralazine-isosorbide dinitrate in the treatment of chronic congestive heart failure. *N Engl J Med.* 1991;325:303-310.

67. Cohn JN, Tognoni G, Glazer RD, Spormann D, Hester A. Rationale and design of the Valsartan Heart Failure Trial: a large multinational trial to assess the effects of valsartan, an angiotensin-receptor blocker, on morbidity and mortality in chronic congestive heart failure. *J Card Fail.* 1999;5:155-160.

68. Cohn JN, Tognoni G; Valsartan Heart Failure Trial Investigators. A randomized trial of the angiotensin-receptor blocker valsartan in chronic heart failure. *N Engl J Med.* 2001;345:1667-1675.

69. Cohn JN, Ziesche S, Smith R, et al. Effect of the calcium antagonist felodipine as supplementary vasodilator therapy in patients with chronic heart failure treated with enalapril. V-HeFT III. Vasodilator-Heart Failure Trial (V-HeFT) Study Group. *Circulation.* 1997;96:856-863.

14

70. Colucci WS, Elkayam U, Horton DP, et al. Intravenous nesiritide, a natriuretic peptide, in the treatment of decompensated heart failure. *N Engl J Med.* 2000;343:246-253.

71. Colucci WS, Packer M, Bristow MR, et al. Carvedilol inhibits clinical progression in patients with mild symptoms of heart failure. US Carvedilol Heart Failure Study Group. *Circulation.* 1996;94:2800-2806.

72. Connolly SJ, Gent M, Roberts RS, et al. Canadian implantable defibrillator study (CIDS): a randomized trial of the implantable cardioverter defibrillator against amiodarone. *Circulation.* 2000;101:1297-1302.

73. Connors AF Jr, Speroff T, Dawson NV, et al. The effectiveness of right heart catheterization in the initial care of critically ill patients. SUPPORT Investigators. *JAMA.* 1996;276:889-897.

74. The CONSENSUS Trial Study Group. Effects of enalapril on mortality in severe congestive heart failure. Results of the Cooperative North Scandinavian Enalapril Survival Study (CONSENSUS). *N Engl J Med* 1987;316:1429-1435.

75. Conti J, Curtis A, Aranda J Jr, Abraham WT, Petersen-Stejskal S, Paulsen D. Are there differences in gender response to cardiac resynchronization therapy? Analysis of the MIRACLE trial. *PACE.* 2002;24:694. Abstract.

76. Crispell KA, Hanson EL, Coates K, Toy W, Hershberger RE. Periodic rescreening is indicated for family members at risk of developing familial dilated cardiomyopathy. *J Am Coll Cardiol.* 2002;39:1503-1507.

77. Cuffe MS, Califf RM, Adams KF Jr, et al. Short term intravenous milrinone for acute exacerbation of chronic heart failure. *JAMA.* 2002;287:1541-1547.

78. Curtis AB, Cannom DS, Bigger JT Jr, et al. Baseline characteristics of patients in the coronary artery bypass graft (CABG) Patch Trial. *Am Heart J.* 1997;134:787-798.

79. Cutler J. Which drug for treatment of hypertension? *Lancet.* 1999;353:604-605.

80. Daoud E, Hummel J, Higgins S, et al. Does ventricular resynchronization therapy influence total survival? *PACE.* 2001;24:539. Abstract.

81. Davies RF, Beanlands DS, Nadeau C, et al. Enalapril versus digoxin in patients with congestive heart failure: a multicenter study. Canadian Enalapril Versus Digoxin Study Group. *J Am Coll Cardiol.* 1991;18:1602-1609.

82. Deedwania PC, Singh BN, Ellenbogen K, Fisher S, Fletcher R, Singh SN. Spontaneous conversion and maintenance of sinus rhythm by amiodarone in patients with heart failure and atrial fibrillation: observations from the veterans affairs congestive heart failure survival trial of antiarrhythmic therapy (CHF-STAT). The Department of Veterans Affairs CHF-STAT Investigators. *Circulation.* 1998;98:2574-2579.

83. Deisenhofer I, Schneider MA, Bohlen-Knauf M, et al. Circumferential mapping and electric isolation of pulmonary veins in patients with atrial fibrillation. *Am J Cardiol.* 2003;91:159-163.

84. Digitalis Investigation Group. The effect of digoxin on mortality and morbidity in patients with heart failure. *N Engl J Med.* 1997;336:525-533.

85. Doughty RN, Whalley GA, Gamble G, MacMahon S, Sharpe N. Left ventricular remodeling with carvedilol in patients with congestive heart failure due to ischemic heart disease. Australia-New Zealand Heart Failure Research Collaborative Group. *J Am Coll Cardiol.* 1997;29:1060-1066.

86. Doval HC, Nul DR, Grancelli HO, Perrone SV, Bortman GR, Curiel R. Randomised trial of low-dose amiodarone in severe congestive heart failure. Grupo de Estudio de la Sobrevida en la Insuficiencia Cardiaca en Argentina (GESICA). *Lancet.* 1994;344:493-498.

87. Dracup K, Baker DW, Dunbar SB, et al. Management of heart failure. II. Counseling, education, and lifestyle modifications. *JAMA.* 1994;272:1442-1446.

88. Eichhorn EJ, Bristow MR. Practical guidelines for initiation of beta-adrenergic blockade in patients with chronic heart failure. *Am J Cardiol.* 1997;79:794-798. Editorial.

89. Etanercept in Congestive Heart Failure. The RENAISSANCE (Randomized Etanercept North American Strategy to Study Antagonism of Cytokines). Trial Handbook. Immunex. Seattle, Wash; 2001.

90. European Coronary Surgery Study Group. Long-term results of prospective randomised study of coronary artery bypass surgery in stable angina pectoris. *Lancet.* 1982;2:1173-1180.

91. Exner DV, Dries DL, Waclawiw MA, Shelton B, Domanski MJ. Beta-adrenergic blocking agent use and mortality in patients with asymptomatic and symptomatic left ventricular systolic dysfunction: a post hoc analysis of the Studies of Left Ventricular Dysfunction. *J Am Coll Cardiol* 1999;33:916-923.

92. Exner DV, Reiffel JA, Epstein AE, et al. Beta-blocker use and survival in patients with ventricular fibrillation or symptomatic ventricular tachycardia: the Antiarrhythmics Versus Implantable Defibrillators (AVID) trial. *J Am Coll Cardiol.* 1999;34:325-333.

14

93. Farquharson CAJ, Struthers AD. Angiotensin II receptor blockers in chronic heart failure—not as ELITE as expected! *J Renin-Angiotensin-Aldosterone Sys.* 2000;1:21-22.

94. Fazio S, Sabatini D, Capaldo B, et al. A preliminary study of growth hormone in the treatment of dilated cardiomyopathy. *N Engl J Med.* 1996;334:809-814.

95. Feldman A, Young JB, Bourge R, et al for the VesT Investigators. Mechanism of increased mortality from vesnarinone in the severe heart failure trial (VesT). *J Am Coll Cardiol.* 1997;29(suppl A):64A.

96. Feldman AM, Bristow MR, Parmley WW, et al. Effects of vesnarinone on morbidity and mortality in patients with heart failure. Vesnarinone Study Group. *N Engl J Med.* 1993;329:149-155.

97. Fonarow GC, Adams KF, Abraham WT, ADHERE Investigators. Risk stratification for in-hospital mortality in heart failure using Classification and Regression Tree (CART) methodology: analysis of 33,046 patients in the ADHERE™ registry. *J Card Fail.* 2003;9(suppl 5):S79. Abstract.

98. Fonarow GC, Chelimsky-Fallick C, Stevenson LW, et al. Effect of direct vasodilation with hydralazine versus angiotensin-converting enzyme inhibition with captopril on mortality in advanced heart failure: the Hy-C trial. *J Am Coll Cardiol.* 1992;19:842-850.

99. Fonarow GC, Stevenson LW, Walden JA, et al. Impact of a comprehensive heart failure management program on hospital readmission and functional status of patients with advanced heart failure. *J Am Coll Cardiol.* 1997;30:725-732.

100. Frazier OH, Delgado RM. Mechanical circulatory support for advanced heart failure: where does it stand in 2003? *Circulation.* 2003;108:3064-3068.

101. Funck-Brentano C, Lancar R, Le Heuzey JY, Lardoux H, Soubrie C, Lechat P. Predictors of medical events in patients enrolled in the cardiac insufficiency bisoprolol study (CIBIS): a study of the interactions between beta-blocker therapy and occurrence of critical events using analysis of competitive risks. *Am Heart J.* 2000;139:262-271.

102. Galley HF. Renal-dose dopamine: will the message now get through? *Lancet.* 2000;356:2112-2113.

103. Gerstenfeld EP, Guerra P, Sparks PB, et al. Clinical outcome after radiofrequency catheter ablation of focal atrial fibrillation triggers. *J Cardiovasc Electrophysiol.* 2001;12:900-908.

104. Gheorghiade M. No effect of amlodipine on mortality or cardiovascular morbidity in patients with severe chronic heart failure. *Evidence-Based Cardiovasc Med.* June, 1997:45.

105. Gheorghiade M, for the OPTIME Investigators. Outcomes of a Prospective Trial of Intravenous Milrinone for Exacerbation of Chronic Heart Failure: OPTIME-CHF. Late-breaking clinical trials. Annual Scientific Sessions. American College of Cardiology, Anaheim, Calif; March 2000.

106. Gheorghiade M, Pitt B. Digitalis Investigation Group (DIG) trial: a stimulus for further research. *Am Heart J.* 1997;134:3-12.

107. Giannuzzi P, Temporelli PL, Corra U, et al. Attenuation of unfavorable remodeling by exercise training in postinfarction patients with left ventricular dysfunction: results of the Exercise in Left Ventricular Dysfunction (ELVD) trial. *Circulation.* 1997;96:1790-1797.

108. Gilbert EM, Abraham WT, Olsen S, et al. Comparative hemodynamic, left ventricular function, and antiadrenergic effects of chronic treatment with metoprolol versus carvedilol in the failing heart. *Circulation.* 1996;94:2817-2825.

109. Granger CB, Ertl G, Kuch J, et al. Randomized trial of candesartan cilexetil in the treatment of patients with congestive heart failure and a history of intolerance to angiotensin-converting enzyme inhibitors. *Am Heart J.* 2000; 139:609-617.

110. Granger CB, McMurray JJ, Yusuf S, et al; CHARM Investigators and Committees. Effects of candesartan in patients with chronic heart failure and reduced left-ventricular systolic function intolerant to angiotensin-converting-enzyme inhibitors: the CHARM-Alternative trial. *Lancet.* 2003; 362:772-776.

111. Greenberg BH. Role of angiotensin receptor blockers in heart failure: not yet RESOLVD. *Circulation.* 1999;100: 1032-1034. Editorial.

112. Grinstead WC, Francis MJ, Marks GF, Tawa CB, Zoghbi WA, Young JB. Discontinuation of chronic diuretic therapy in stable congestive heart failure secondary to coronary artery disease or to idiopathic dilated cardiomyopathy. *Am J Cardiol.* 1994;73:881-886.

113. Guidelines for the evaluation and management of heart failure. Committee on Evaluation and Management of Heart Failure. Report of the American College of Cardiology/American Heart Association Task Force on Practice Guidelines. *J Am Coll Cardiol.* 1995;26:1376-1398.

114. Haissaguerre M, Jais P, Shah DC, et al. Electrophysiological end point for catheter ablation of atrial fibrillation initiated from multiple pulmonary venous foci. *Circulation.* 2000;101:1409-1417.

14

115. Haissaguerre M, Jais P, Shah DC, et al. Right and left atrial radiofrequency catheter therapy of paroxysmal atrial fibrillation. *J Cardiovasc Electrophysiol*. 1996;7:1132-1144.

116. Haisaguerre M, Jais P, Shah DC, et al. Spontaneous initiation of atrial fibrillation by ectopic beats originating in the pulmonary veins. *N Engl J Med*. 1998;339:659-666.

117. Haissaguerre M, Shah DC, Jais P, et al. Electrophysiological breakthroughs from the left atrium to the pulmonary veins. *Circulation*. 2000;102:2463-2465.

118. Hall AS, Murray GD, Ball SG. Follow-up study of patients randomly allocated ramipril or placebo for heart failure after acute myocardial infarction: AIRE Extension (AIREX) Study. Acute Infarction Ramipril Efficacy. *Lancet*. 1997;349:1493-1497.

119. Hallstrom A, Pratt CM, Greene HL, et al. Relations between heart failure, ejection fraction, arrhythmia suppression and mortality: analysis of the Cardiac Arrhythmia Suppression Trial. *J Am Coll Cardiol*. 1995;25:1250-1257.

120. Hamer AW, Arkles LB, Johns JA. Beneficial effects of low dose amiodarone in patients with congestive cardiac failure: a placebo-controlled trial. *J Am Coll Cardiol*. 1989;14:1768-1774.

121. Hampton JR, van Veldhuisen DJ, Kleber FX, et al. Randomised study of effect of ibopamine on survival in patients with advanced severe heart failure. Second Prospective Randomised Study of Ibopamine on Mortality and Efficacy (PRIME II) Investigators. *Lancet*. 1997;349:971-977.

122. Hansson L, Lindholm LH, Niskanen L, et al. Effect of angiotensin-converting-enzyme inhibition compared with conventional therapy on cardiovascular morbidity and mortality in hypertension: the Captopril Prevention Project (CAPPP) randomised trial. *Lancet*. 1999;353:611-616.

123. Hanumanthu S, Butler J, Chomsky D, et al. Effect of a heart failure program on hospitalization frequency and exercise tolerance. *Circulation*. 1997;96:2842-2848.

124. Heart Outcomes Prevention Evaluation Study. The design of a large, simple randomized trial of an angiotensin-converting enzyme inhibitor (ramipril) and vitamin E in patients at high risk of cardiovascular events. *Can J Cardiol*. 1996;12:127-137.

125. Heart Outcomes Prevention Evaluation Study Investigators. Effects of ramipril on cardiovascular and microvascular outcomes in people with diabetes mellitus: results of the HOPE study and MICRO-HOPE substudy. *Lancet*. 2000;355:253-259.

126. Heart Outcomes Prevention Evaluation Study Investigators. Yusuf S, Dagenais G, Pogue J, Bosch, J, Sleight P. Vitamin E supplementation and cardiovascular events in high-risk patients. *N Engl J Med*. 2000;342:154-160.

127. Heart Outcomes Prevention Evaluation Study Investigators. Yusuf S, Sleight P, Pogue J, Bosch J, Davies R, Dagenais G. Effects of an angiotensin-converting-enzyme inhibitor, ramipril, on cardiovascular events in high-risk patients. *N Engl J Med.* 2000;342:145-153.

128. Hinkle LE Jr, Thaler HT. Clinical classification of cardiac deaths. *Circulation.* 1982;65:457-464.

129. Hjalmarson A, Goldstein S, Fagerberg B, et al. Effects of controlled-release metoprolol on total mortality, hospitalizations, and well-being in patients with heart failure: the Metoprolol CR/XL Randomized Intervention Trial in congestive heart failure (MERIT-HF). MERIT-HF Study Group. *JAMA.* 2000;283:1295-1302.

130. Hobbs RE, Miller LW, Bott-Silverman C, et al. Hemodynamic effects of a single intravenous injection of synthetic human brain natriuretic peptide in patients with heart failure secondary to ischemic or idiopathic dilated cardiomyopathy. *Am J Cardiol.* 1996;78:896-901.

131. Hochman JS, Sleeper LA, Godfrey E, et al. Should weeEmergently revascularize occluded coronaries for cardiogenic shock: an international randomized trial of emergency PTCA/CABG-trial design. The SHOCK Trial Study Group. *Am Heart J.* 1999;137:313-321.

132. Hochman JS, Sleeper LA, Webb JG, et al. Early revascularization in acute myocardial infarction complicated by cardiogenic shock. SHOCK Investigators. Should We Emergently Revascularize Occluded Coronaries for Cardiogenic Shock. *N Engl J Med.* 1999;341:625-634.

133. Hochman JS, Sleeper LA, White HD, et al. One-year survival following early revascularization for cardiogenic shock. *JAMA.* 2001;285:190-192.

134. Hohnloser SH, Kuck KH, Lilienthal J. Rhythm or rate control in atrial fibrillation—Pharmacological Intervention in Atrial Fibrillation (PIAF): a randomised trial. *Lancet.* 2000;356:1789-1794.

135. Hotline Sessions of the 23rd European Congress of Cardiology. *Eur Heart J.* 2001;22:2033-2037.

136. Israel CW, Hugl B, Unterberg C, et al, for the AT500 Verification Study. Pace-termination and pacing for prevention of atrial tachyarrhythmias: results from a multicenter study with an implantable device for atrial therapy. *J Cardiovasc Electrophysiol.* 2001;12:1121-1128.

137. Jaagosild P, Dawson NV, Thomas C, et al. Outcomes of acute exacerbation of severe congestive heart failure: quality of life, resource use, and survival. SUPPORT Investigators. The Study to Understand Prognosis and Preferences for Outcomes and Risks of Treatments. *Arch Intern Med.* 1998;158:1081-1089.

14

138. Jafri SM, Cleland J, Massie B. Is there a role for warfarin or aspirin therapy in heart failure? *Heart Fail Rev.* 1997;1:271-276.

139. Jafri SM, Mammen EF, Masura J, Goldstein S. Effects of warfarin on markers of hypercoagulability in patients with heart failure. *Am Heart J.* 1997;134:27-36.

140. Jancin B. Major heart failure study halted after 53 deaths: investigators baffled by moxonidine effect. *Intern Med News.* Oct, 1999;32:1-2.

141. Johnson W, Omland T, Hall C, et al. Neurohormonal activation rapidly decreases after intravenous therapy with diuretics and vasodilators for class IV heart failure. *J Am Coll Cardiol.* 2002;39:1623-1629.

142. Julian DG, Camm AJ, Frangin G, et al. Randomised trial of effect of amiodarone on mortality in patients with left-ventricular dysfunction after recent myocardial infarction: EMIAT. European Myocardial Infarct Amiodarone Trial Investigators. *Lancet.* 1997;349:667-674.

143. Kalra PR, Moon JC, Coats AJ. Do results of the ENABLE (Endothelian Antagonist Bosentan for Lowering Cardiac Events in Heart Failure) study spell the end for non-selective endothelin antagonism in heart failure? *Int J Cardiol.* 2002;85:195-197.

144. Kanagaratnam L, Tomassoni G, Schweikert R, et al. Empirical pulmonary vein isolation in patients with chronic atrial fibrillation using a three-dimensional nonfluoroscopic mapping system: long-term follow-up. *Pacing Clin Electrophysiol.* 2001;24:1774-1779.

145. Kanuru NK, DeLurgio DB, Ransom S, et al. Right ventricular septal versus right ventricular apical pacing in biventricular pacing systems does not affect patient functional improvement. *PACE.* 2002;24:648. Abstract.

146. Kasper EK, Gerstenblith G, Hefter G, et al. A randomized trial of the efficacy of multidisciplinary care in heart failure outpatients at high risk of hospital readmission. *J Am Coll Cardiol.* 2002;39:471-480.

147. Khot UN, Novaro GM, Popovic ZB, et al. Nitroprusside in critically ill patients with left ventricular dysfunction and aortic stenosis. *N Engl J Med.* 2003;348:1756-1763.

148. Kjoller-Hansen L, Steffensen R, Grande P. The Angiotensin-converting Enzyme Inhibition Post Revascularization Study (APRES). *J Am Coll Cardiol.* 2000;35:881-888.

149. Kleber FX, Niemoller L, Doering W. Impact of converting enzyme inhibition on progression of chronic heart failure: results of the Munich Mild Heart Failure Trial. *Br Heart J.* 1992;67:289-296.

150. Kober L, Bloch Thomsen PE, Moller M, et al. Effect of dofetilide in patients with recent myocardial infarction and left-ventricular dysfunction: a randomised trial. *Lancet.* 2000;356:2052-2058.

151. Kober L, Torp-Pedersen C, Carlsen JE, et al. A clinical trial of the angiotensin-converting-enzyme inhibitor trandolapril in patients with left ventricular dysfunction after myocardial infarction. Trandolapril Cardiac Evaluation (TRACE) Study Group. *N Engl J Med.* 1995;333:1670-1676.

152. Konstam M, Dracup K, Baker D, et al. Heart failure: evaluation and care of patient with left-ventricular systolic dysfunction. Clinical practice guidelines. AHCPR publication no. 94-0612. Rockville, Md: Agency for Health Care Policy and Research, Public Heart Service, US Department of Health and Human Services; June 1994. Abstract.

153. Konstam MA, Patten RD, Thomas I, et al. Effects of losartan and captopril on left ventricular volumes in elderly patients with heart failure: results of the ELITE ventricular function substudy. *Am Heart J.* 2000;139:1081-1087.

154. Kostis JB, Davis BR, Cutler J, et al. Prevention of heart failure by antihypertensive drug treatment in older persons with isolated systolic hypertension. SHEP Cooperative Research Group. *JAMA.* 1997;278:212-216.

155. Kostis JB, Shelton B, Gosselin G, et al. Adverse effects of enalapril in the Studies of Left Ventricular Dysfunction (SOLVD). SOLVD Investigators. *Am Heart J.* 1996;131: 350-355.

156. Krumholz HM. Beta-blockers for mild to moderate heart failure. *Lancet.* 1999;353:2-3.

157. Krumholz HM, Amatruda J, Smith GL, et al. Randomized trial of an education and support intervention to prevent readmission of patients with heart failure. *J Am Coll Cardiol.* 2002;39:83-89.

158. Kuck KH, Cappato R, Siebels J, Ruppel R. Randomized comparison of antiarrhythmic drug therapy with implantable defibrillators in patients resuscitated from cardiac arrest: the Cardiac Arrest Study Hamburg (CASH). *Circulation.* 2000;102:748-754.

159. Lasagna L. Diuretics vs alpha-blockers for treatment of hypertension: lessons from ALLHAT. Antihypertensive and Lipid-Lowering Treatment to Prevent Heart Attack Trial. *JAMA.* 2000;283:2013-2014. Editorial.

160. Lechat P, Escolano S, Golmard JL, et al. Prognostic value of bisoprolol-induced hemodynamic effects in heart failure during the Cardiac Insufficiency Bisoprolol Study (CIBIS). *Circulation.* 1997;96:2197-2205.

14

161. Leclercq C, Kass DA. Retiming the failing heart: principles and current clinical status of cardiac resynchronization. *J Am Coll Cardiol.* 2002;39:194-201.

162. Leclercq C, Linde C, Cazeau S, et al. Sustained clinical efficacy of biventricular pacing in patients with advanced heart failure and stable sinus rhythm. 2 year follow-up from the MUSTIC study. *PACE (II).* 2002;24:601. Abstract.

163. Lee MA, Weachter R, Pollak S, et al. Can preventive and antitachycardia pacing reduce the frequency and burden of atrial tachyarrhythmias? The ATTEST study results. *Pacing Clin Electrophysiol.* 2002;25:541. Abstract 74.

164. Lenfant C. JNC guidelines: is the message getting through? Joint National Commission on Detection, Evaluation, and Treatment of High Blood Pressure. *JAMA.* 1997;278:1778-1779. Editorial.

165. Leon AR, Brozena S, Liang CS, et al. Effect of cardiac resynchronization therapy with sequential biventricular pacing on Doppler-derived left ventricular stroke volume, functional status and exercise capacity in patients with ventricular dysfunction and conduction delay: the US InSync III trial. *PACE.* 2002;24:558. Abstract.

166. Levine TB, Bernink PJ, Caspi A, et al. Effect of mibefradil, a T-type calcium channel blocker, on morbidity and mortality in moderate to severe congestive heart failure: the MACH-1 study. Mortality Assessment in Congestive Heart Failure Trial. *Circulation.* 2000;101:758-764.

167. Levy D, Kenchaiah S, Larson MG, et al. Long-term trends in the incidence of and survival with heart failure. *N Engl J Med.* 2002;347:1397-1402.

168. Liem L, Leon A, Young JB. Effectiveness of bi-ventricular antitachycardia pacing in CHF patients receiving cardiac resynchronization therapy. *PACE.* 2002;24:647. Abstract.

169. Linde C, Leclercq C, Rex S, et al. Long-term benefits of biventricular pacing in congestive heart failure: results from the Multisite Stimulation in Cardiomyopathy (MUSTIC) study. *J Am Coll Cardiol.* 2002;40:111-118.

170. Lloyd-Jones DM, Larson MG, Leip EP, et al; Framingham Heart Study. Lifetime risk for developing congestive heart failure: the Framingham Heart Study. *Circulation.* 2002;106:3068-3072.

171. Loh E, Swain JL. Growth hormone for heart failure—cause for cautious optimism. *N Engl J Med.* 1996;334:856-857. Editorial.

172. Lonn E, Yusuf S, Dzavik V, et al. Effects of ramipril and vitamin E on atherosclerosis: the study to evaluate carotid ultrasound changes in patients treated with ramipril and vitamin E (SECURE). *Circulation.* 2001;103:919-925.

173. Macle L, Jais P, Weerasooriya R, et al. Irrigated-tip catheter ablation of pulmonary veins for treatment of atrial fibrillation. *J Cardiovasc Electrophysiol.* 2002;13:1067-1073.

174. Madsen EB, Gilpin E, Henning H, et al. Prognostic importance of digitalis after acute myocardial infarction. *J Am Coll Cardiol.* 1984;3:681-689.

175. Mahmarian JJ, Smart FW, Moye LA, et al. Exploring the minimal dose of amiodarone with antiarrhythmic and hemodynamic activity. *Am J Cardiol.* 1994;74:681-686.

176. Maisel A. B-Type natriuretic peptide in the diagnosis and management of congestive heart failure. *Cardiol Clin.* 2001;19:557-571.

177. Maisel A. B-Type natriuretic peptide levels: diagnostic and prognostic in congestive heart failure. What's next? *Circulation.* 2002;105:2328-2331. Editorial.

178. Makin EJB. Zambon Corporation. ESPRIT Study Update. Personal communication. November 1, 1995.

179. Mangrum JM, Mounsey JP, Kok LC, et al. Intracardiac echocardiography-guided, anatomically based radiofrequency ablation of focal atrial fibrillation originating from pulmonary veins. *J Am Coll Cardiol.* 2002;39:1964-1972.

180. Mark DB, Felker GM. B-type natriuretic peptide–a biomarker for all seasons? *N Engl J Med.* 2004;350:718-720.

181. Marrouche NF, Dresing T, Cole C, et al. Circular mapping and ablation of the pulmonary vein for treatment of atrial fibrillation: impact of different catheter technologies. *J Am Coll Cardiol.* 2002;40:464-474.

182. Marrouche NF, Martin DO, Wazni O, et al. Phased-array intracardiac echocardiography monitoring during pulmonary vein isolation in patients with atrial fibrillation: impact on outcome and complications. *Circulation.* 2003;107:2710-2716.

183. Mason JW, O'Connell JB, Herskowitz A, et al. A clinical trial of immunosuppressive therapy for myocarditis. The Myocarditis Treatment Trial Investigators. *N Engl J Med.* 1995;333:269-275.

184. Massie BM, Berk MR, Brozena SC, et al. Can further benefit be achieved by adding flosequinan to patients with congestive heart failure who remain symptomatic on diuretic, digoxin, and an angiotensin converting enzyme inhibitor? Results of the Flosequinan-ACE inhibitor Trial (FACET). *Circulation.* 1993;88:492-501.

185. McCarthy PM, Gillinov AM, Castle L, et al. The Cox–Maze procedure: the Cleveland Clinic experience. *Semin Thorac Cardiovasc Surg.* 2000;12:25-29.

186. McCullough PA, Nowak RM, McCord J, et al. B-type natriuretic peptide and clinical judgment in emergency diagnosis of heart failure: analysis from Breathing Not Properly (BNP) Multinational Study. *Circulation.* 2002;106:416-422.

14

187. McKelvie RS, Rouleau JL, White M, et al. Comparative impact of enalapril, candesartan or metoprolol alone or in combination on ventricular remodelling in patients with congestive heart failure. *Eur Heart J.* 2003;24:1727-1734.

188. McKelvie RS, Yusuf S, Pericak D, et al. Comparison of candesartan, enalapril, and their combination in congestive heart failure: randomized evaluation of strategies for left ventricular dysfunction (RESOLVD) pilot study. The RESOLVD Pilot Study Investigators. *Circulation.* 1999;100:1056-1064.

189. McMurray JJ, Ostergren J, Swedberg K, et al; CHARM Investigators and Committees. Effects of candesartan in patients with chronic heart failure and reduced left-ventricular systolic function taking angiotensin-converting-enzyme inhibitors: the CHARM-Added trial. *Lancet.* 2003;362:767-771.

190. McNamara DM, Starling RC, Dec WG, et al. Intervention in myocarditis and acute cardiomyopathy with immune globulin: results of the placebo controlled IMAC trial. *Circulation.* 2001;103:2254-2259.

191. MERIT-HF Study Group. Effect of metoprolol CR/XL in chronic heart failure: Metoprolol CR/XL Randomised Intervention Trial in Congestive Heart Failure. *Lancet.* 1999;353:2001-2007.

192. Mills RM, LeJemtel TH, Horton DP, et al. Sustained hemodynamic effects of an infusion of nesiritide (human B-type natriuretic peptide) in heart failure. *J Am Coll Cardiol.* 1999;34:155-162.

193. MIRACLE-ICD Trial Handbook. Medtronic, Inc. Minneapolis, Minn; 2001.

194. Mittal S, Iwai S, Stein KM, Markowitz SM, Slotwiner DJ, Lerman BB. Long-term outcome of patients with unexplained syncope treated with an electrophysiologic-guided approach in the implantable cardioverter-defibrillator era. *J Am Coll Cardiol.* 1999;34:1082-1098.

195. Moe GW, Rouleau JL, Charbonneau L, et al. Neurohormonal activation in severe heart failure: relation to patient death and the effect of treatment with flosequinan. *Am Heart J.* 2000;139:587-595.

196. Moore J. Do HOPE results mean all high-risk patients should take ACE inhibitors? *Cardiology Today.* February, 2001:9.

197. Moss AJ, Davis HT, Conard DL, De Camilla JJ, Odoroff CL. Digitalis-associated cardiac mortality after myocardial infarction. *Circulation.* 1981;64:1150-1156.

198. Moss AJ, Hall WJ, Cannom DS, et al. Improved survival with an implanted defibrillator in patients with coronary disease at high risk for ventricular arrhythmia. Multicenter Automatic Defibrillator Implantation Trial Investigators. *N Engl J Med.* 1996;335:1933-1940.

199. Moss AJ, Zareba W, Hall WJ, et al. Prophylactic implantation of a defibrillator in patients with myocardial infarction and reduced ejection fraction. *N Engl J Med.* 2002;346:877-883.

200. Mueller C, Scholer A, Laule-Kilian K, et al. Use of B-type natriuretic peptide in the evaluation and management of acute dyspnea. *N Engl J Med.* 2004;350:647-654.

201. Myerburg RJ, Castellanos A. Clinical trials of implantable defibrillators. *New Engl J Med.* 1997;337:1621-1623. Editorial.

202. Natale A, Pisano E, Shewchik J, et al. First human experience with pulmonary vein isolation using a through-the-balloon circumferential ultrasound ablation system for recurrent atrial fibrillation. *Circulation.* 2000;102:1879-1882.

203. Nozba MM, Boskis B, Bristow M, et al. WHO concise guide to the management of heart failure. *J Cardiac Failure.* 1996;2:153-155.

204. Oral H, Knight BP, Ozaydin M, et al. Segmental ostial ablation to isolate the pulmonary veins during atrial fibrillation: feasibility and mechanistic insights. *Circulation.* 2002;106:1256-1262.

205. Oral H, Knight BP, Tada H, et al. Pulmonary vein isolation for paroxysmal and persistent atrial fibrillation. *Circulation.* 2002;105:1077-1081.

206. Packer M. ACTION heart failure treatment guidelines. *Am J Cardiol.* 1999;83:1-110.

207. Packer M. Effects of phosphodiesterase inhibitors on survival of patients with chronic congestive heart failure. *Am J Cardiol.* 1989;63:41A-45A.

208. Packer M. Effects of the Endothelin Receptor Antagonist Bosartan on Morbidity and Mortality in Patients With Chronic Heart Failure: Results of the ENABLE 1 and 2 Trial Programs. Presented at the 51st Annual Scientific Sessions of the American College of Cardiology, Atlanta, Ga. March, 2002.

209. Packer M. End of the oldest controversy in medicine. Are we ready to conclude the debate on digitalis? *N Engl J Med.* 1997;336:575-576. Editorial.

210. Packer M, Bristow MR, Cohn JN, et al. The effect of carvedilol on morbidity and mortality in patients with chronic heart failure. US Carvedilol Heart Failure Study Group. *N Engl J Med.* 1996;334:1349-1355.

211. Packer M, Califf RM, Konstam MA, et al. Comparison of omapatrilat and enalapril in patients with chronic heart failure: the Omapatrilat Versus Enalapril Randomized Trial of Utility in Reducing Events (OVERTURE). *Circulation.* 2002;106:920-926.

14

212. Packer M, Carver JR, Rodeheffer RJ, et al. Effect of oral milrinone on mortality in severe chronic heart failure. The PROMISE Study Research Group. *N Engl J Med.* 1991;325:1468-1475.

213. Packer M, Coats AJS, Fowler MB, et al. Effect of carvedilol on survival in severe chronic heart failure. *N Engl J Med.* 2001;344:1651-1658.

214. Packer M, Colucci WS, Sackner-Bernstein JD, et al. Double-blind, placebo-controlled study of the effects of carvedilol in patients with moderate to severe heart failure. The PRE-CISE Trial. Prospective Randomized Evaluation of Carvedilol on Symptoms and Exercise. *Circulation.* 1996;94:2793-2799.

215. Packer M, Gheorghiade M, Young JB, et al. Withdrawal of digoxin from patients with chronic heart failure treated with angiotensin-converting-enzyme inhibitors. RADIANCE Study. *N Engl J Med.* 1993;329:1-7.

216. Packer M, Narahara KA, Elkayam U, et al. Double-blind, placebo-controlled study of the efficacy of flosequinan in patients with chronic heart failure. Principal Investigators of the RE-FLECT Study. *J Am Coll Cardiol.* 1993;22:65-72.

217. Packer M, O'Connor CM, Ghali JK, et al. Effect of amlodipine on morbidity and mortality in severe chronic heart failure. Prospective Randomized Amlodipine Survival Evaluation Study Group. *N Engl J Med.* 1996;335:1107-1114.

218. Packer M, Poole-Wilson PA, Armstrong PW, et al. Comparative effects of low and high doses of the angiotensin-converting enzyme inhibitor, lisinopril, on morbidity and mortality in chronic heart failure. ATLAS Study Group. *Circulation.* 1999;100:2312-2318.

219. Padeletti L, Pieragnoli P, Ciapetti C, et al. Randomized crossover comparison of right atrial appendage pacing versus interatrial septum pacing for prevention of paroxysmal atrial fibrillation in patients with sinus bradycardia. *Am Heart J.* 2001;142:1047-1055.

220. Padeletti L, Purerfellner H, Adler S, et al. Atrial septal lead placement and atrial pacing algorithms for prevention of paroxysmal atrial fibrillation: ASPECT study results. *Pacing Clin Electrophysiol.* 2002;25:687. Abstract 659.

221. Pagel PS, Haikala H, Pentikainen PJ, et al. Pharmacology of levosimendan: a new myofilament calcium sensitizer. *Cardiovasc Drug Rev.* 1996;14:286-316.

222. Pagley PR, Beller GA, Watson DD, Gimple LW, Ragosta M. Improved outcome after coronary bypass surgery in patients with ischemic cardiomyopathy and residual myocardial viability. *Circulation.* 1997;96:793-800.

223. Pappone C, Oreto G, Rosanio S, et al. Atrial electroanatomic remodeling after circumferential radiofrequency pulmonary vein ablation. *Circulation.* 2001;104:2539-2544.

224. Pappone C, Rosanio S, Oreto G, et al. Circumferential radiofrequency ablation of pulmonary vein ostia: a new anatomic approach for curing atrial fibrillation. *Circulation.* 2000;102:2619-2628.

225. Parmley WW. Clinical practice guidelines. Does the cookbook have enough recipes? *JAMA.* 1994;272:1374-1375. Editorial.

226. Persson H, Rythe'n-Alder E, Melcher A, Erhardt L. Effects of beta receptor antagonists in patients with clinical evidence of heart failure after myocardial infarction: double blind comparison of metoprolol and xamoterol. *Br Heart J.* 1995;74:140-148.

227. Pfeffer MA, Braunwald E, Moye LA, et al. Effect of captopril on mortality and morbidity in patients with left ventricular dysfunction after myocardial infarction. Results of the survival and ventricular enlargement trial. The SAVE Investigators. *N Engl J Med.* 1992;327:669-677.

228. Pfeffer MA, McMurray JJ, Velazquez EJ, et al; Valsartan in Acute Myocardial Infarction Trial Investigators. Valsartan, captopril, or both in myocardial infarction complicated by heart failure, left ventricular dysfunction, or both. *N Engl J Med.* 2003;349:1893-1906.

229. Pfeffer MA, Swedberg K, Granger CB, et al; CHARM Investigators and Committees. Effects of candesartan on mortality and morbidity in patients with chronic heart failure: the CHARM-Overall programme. *Lancet.* 2003;362:759-766.

230. Pimobendan in Congestive Heart Failure (PICO) Investigators. Effect of pimobendan on exercise capacity in patients with heart failure: main results from the Pimobendan in Congestive Heart Failure (PICO) trial. *Heart.* 1996;76:223-231.

231. Pitt B, Chang P, Timmermans PB. Angiotensin II receptor antagonists in heart failure: rationale and design of the Evaluation of Losartan in the Elderly (ELITE) trial. *Cardiovasc Drugs Ther.* 1995;9:693-700.

232. Pitt B, Poole-Wilson P, Segal R, et al. Effects of losartan versus captopril on mortality in patients with symptomatic heart failure: rationale, design, and baseline characteristics of patients in the Losartan Heart Failure Survival Study—ELITE II. *J Card Fail.* 1999;5:146-154.

233. Pitt B, Remme W, Zannad F, et al; Eplerenone Post-Acute Myocardial Infarction Heart Failure Efficacy and Survival Study Investigators. Eplerenone, a selective aldosterone blocker, in patients with left ventricular dysfunction after myocardial infarction. *N Engl J Med.* 2003;348:1309-1321.

14

234. Pitt B, Segal R, Martinez FA, et al. Randomised trial of losartan versus captopril in patients over 65 with heart failure (Evaluation of Losartan in the Elderly Study, ELITE). *Lancet.* 1997;349:747-752.

235. Pitt B, Williams G, Remme W, et al. The EPHESUS trial: eplerenone in patients with heart failure due to systolic dysfunction complicating acute myocardial infarction. Eplerenone Post-AMI Heart Failure Efficacy and Survival Study. *Cardiovasc Drugs Ther.* 2001;15:79-87.

236. Pitt B, Zannad F, Remme WJ, et al. The effect of spironolactone on morbidity and mortality in patients with severe heart failure. Randomized Aldactone Evaluation Study Investigators. *N Engl J Med.* 1999;341:709-717.

237. Podrid PJ. Amiodarone: reevaluation of an old drug. *Ann Intern Med.* 1995;122:689-700.

238. Poole-Wilson PA, Swedberg K, Cleland JGF, et al. Comparison of carvedilol and metoprolol on clinical outcomes in patients with chronic heart failure in the Carvedilol Or Metoprolol European Trial (COMET): randomised controlled trial. *Lancet.* 2003;362:7-13.

239. The Post Coronary Artery Bypass Graft Trial Investigators. The effect of aggressive lowering of low-density lipoprotein cholesterol levels and low-dose anticoagulation on obstructive changes in saphenous-vein coronary-artery bypass grafts. *N Engl J Med.* 1997;336:153-162.

240. Pratt CM, Eaton T, Francis M, et al. The inverse relationship between baseline left ventricular ejection fraction and outcome of antiarrhythmic therapy: a dangerous imbalance in the risk-benefit ratio. *Am Heart J.* 1989;118:433-440.

241. Pratt CM, Francis M, Mahler S, Aogaichi K, Keus P, Young JB. The natural history of benign and potentially malignant ventricular arrhythmias with special reference to nonsustained ventricular tachycardia. *Am Heart J.* 1988;116:897-903.

242. PROFILE Investigators Group. Prospective randomized flosequinan longevity evaluation. *Circulation.* 1993;88 (suppl 1):1-301. Abstract.

243. Psaty BM, Smith NL, Siscovick DS, et al. Health outcomes associated with antihypertensive therapies used as first-line agents. A systematic review and meta-analysis. *JAMA.* 1997;277:739-745.

244. Publication Committee for the VMAC Investigators. Intravenous nesiritide versus nitroglycerin for treatment of decompensated congestive heart failure. *JAMA.* 2002;287:1531-1540.

245. Qin JX, Shiota T, McCarthy PM, et al. Importance of mitral valve repair associated with left ventricular reconstruction for patients with ischemic cardiomyopathy: a real-time three-dimensional echocardiographic study. *Circulation.* 2003;108(suppl 1):II241-II246.

246. Rauh RA, Schwabauer NJ, Enger EL, Moran JF. A community hospital-based congestive heart failure program: impact on length of stay, admission and readmission rates and cost. *Am J Manage Care.* 1999;5:37-43.

247. Redfors A. Plasma digoxin concentration—its relation to digoxin dosage and clinical effects in patients with atrial fibrillation. *Br Heart J.* 1972;34:383-391.

248. RESOLVD Investigators. Effects of metoprolol CR in patients with ischemic and dilated cardiomyopathy: the randomized evaluation of strategies for left ventricular dysfunction pilot study. *Circulation.* 2000;101:378-384.

249. Rich MW, Beckham V, Wittenberg C, Leven CL, Freedland KE, Carney RM. A multidisciplinary intervention to prevent the readmission of elderly patients with congestive heart failure. *N Engl J Med.* 1995;333:1190-1195.

250. Rich MW, Gray DB, Beckham V, Wittenberg C, Luther P. Effect of a multidisciplinary intervention on medication compliance in elderly patients with congestive heart failure. *Am J Med.* 1996;101:270-276.

251. Richards AM, Nicholls MG. Aldosterone antagonism in heart failure. *Lancet.* 1999;354:789-790.

252. Riegger GA, Bouzo H, Petr P, et al. Improvement in exercise tolerance and symptoms of congestive heart failure during treatment with candesartan cilexetil. Symptom, Tolerability, Response to Exercise Trial of Candesartan Cilexetil in Heart Failure (STRETCH) Investigators. *Circulation.* 1999;100:2224-2230.

253. Rodkey SM, Young JB. The cardiovascular use of diuretics. *Card Clin N Am.* 1997;1:63-80.

254. Rose EA, Gelijns AC, Moskowitz AJ, et al. Long-term mechanical left ventricular assistance for end-stage heart failure. *N Engl J Med.* 2001;345:1435-1443.

255. Rouleau JL, Pfeffer MA, Stewart DJ, et al. Comparison of vasopeptidase inhibitor, omapatrilat, and lisinopril on exercise tolerance and morbidity in patients with heart failure: IMPRESS randomised trial. *Lancet.* 2000;356:615-620.

256. Saliba W, Wilber D, Packer D, et al. Circumferential ultrasound ablation for pulmonary vein isolation: analysis of acute and chronic failures. *J Cardiovasc Electrophysiol.* 2002;13:957-961.

257. Sanders P, Morton JB, Deen VR, et al. Immediate and long-term results of radiofrequency ablation of pulmonary vein ectopy for cure of paroxysmal atrial fibrillation using a focal approach. *Intern Med J.* 2002;32:202-207.

258. Seidl K, Cazeau S, Gaita F, et al. Dual-site pacing vs monosite pacing in prevention of atrial fibrillation. *Pacing Clin Electrophysiol.* 2002;24:568. Abstract 184.

14

259. Shah MR, Granger CB, Bart BA, et al. Sex-related differences in the use and adverse effects of angiotensin-converting enzyme inhibitors in heart failure: the study of patients intolerant of converting enzyme inhibitors registry. *Am J Med.* 2000;109:489-492.

260. Shah MR, O'Connor CM, Sopko G, Hasslebland V, Califf RM, Stevenson LW, for the ESCAPE investigators. Evaluation Study of Congestive Heart Failure and Pulmonary Artery Catheterization Effectiveness (ESCAPE): design and rationale. *Am Heart J.* 2001;141:528-535.

261. Sharpe N. Benefit of beta-blockers for heart failure: proven in 1999. *Lancet.* 1999;353:1988-1989.

262. Sharpe N. High-dose lisinopril was efficacious and safe in reducing the risk of death and hospitalization in chronic heart failure. *Evidence-Based Cardiovasc Med.* 2000;4:44.

263. Sheldon R, Connolly S, Krahn A, Roberts R, Gent M, Gardner M. Identification of patients most likely to benefit from implantable cardioverter-defibrillator therapy: the Canadian Implantable Defibrillator Study. *Circulation.* 2000;101:1660-1664.

264. Shenkman HJ, Pampati V, Khandelwal AK, et al. Congestive heart failure and QRS duration: establishing prognosis study. *Chest.* 2002;122:528-534.

265. Siegel D, Lopez J. Trends in antihypertensive drug use in the United States: do the JNC V recommendations affect prescribing? Fifth Joint National Commission on the Detection, Evaluation, and Treatment of High Blood Pressure. *JAMA.* 1997;278:1745-1748.

266. Silke B. Central hemodynamic effects of diuretic therapy in chronic heart failure. *Cardiovasc Drugs Ther.* 1993;7(suppl 1):45-53.

267. Silke B. Haemodynamic impact of diuretic therapy in chronic heart failure. *Cardiology.* 1994;84(suppl 2):115-123.

268. Silver MJ, Young J, Topol EJ. Amiodarone in congestive heart failure. *N Engl J Med.* 1995;333:1639-1640. Letter.

269. Sim I, McDonald KM, Lavori PW, Norbutas CM, Hlatky MA. Quantitative overview of randomized trials of amiodarone to prevent sudden cardiac death. *Circulation.* 1997;96:2823-2829.

270. Singh SN, Fletcher RD, Fisher S, et al. Veterans Affairs congestive heart failure antiarrhythmic trial. CHF STAT Investigators. *Am J Cardiol.* 1993;72:99F-102F.

271. Singh SN, Fletcher RD, Fisher SG, et al. Amiodarone in patients with congestive heart failure and asymptomatic ventricular arrhythmia. Survival Trial of Antiarrhythmic Therapy in Congestive Heart Failure. *N Engl J Med.* 1995;333:77-82.

272. The Sixth Report of the Joint National Committee on Prevention, Detection, Evaluation, and Treatment of High Blood Pressure. *Arch Intern Med.* 1997;157:2413-2446.

273. Slatton ML, Irani WN, Hall SA, et al. Does digoxin provide additional hemodynamic and autonomic benefit at higher doses in patients with mild to moderate heart failure and normal sinus rhythm? *J Am Coll Cardiol.* 1997;29:1206-1213.

274. Sleight P. The HOPE study (Heart Outcomes Prevention Evaluation). *J Renin-Angiotensin-Aldosterone Sys.* 2000;1:18-20.

275. Smith TW. Digoxin in heart failure. *N Engl J Med.* 1993;329:51-53. Editorial.

276. The SOLVD Investigators. Effect of enalapril on mortality and the development of heart failure in asymptomatic patients with reduced left ventricular ejection fractions. *N Engl J Med.* 1992;327:685-691.

277. The SOLVD Investigators. Effect of enalapril on survival in patients with reduced left ventricular ejection fractions and congestive heart failure. *N Engl J Med.* 1991;325:293-302.

278. The SOLVD Investigators. Studies of left ventricular dysfunction (SOLVD)—rationale, design and methods: two trials that evaluate the effect of enalapril in patients with reduced ejection fraction. *Am J Cardiol.* 1990;66:315-322.

279. Starling RC, Young JB, Scalia GM, et al. Preliminary observations with ventricular remodeling surgery for refractory congestive heart failure. *J Am Coll Cardiol.* 1997;29:5A-64A.

280. Stewart S, Marley JE, Horowitz JD. Effects of a multidisciplinary, home-based intervention on unplanned readmissions and survival among patients with chronic congestive heart failure: a randomized controlled study. *Lancet.* 1999;354:1077-1083.

281. St. John Sutton M, Kokovic D, Plappert T, et al. Cardiac resynchronization therapy results in reverse remodeling in both ischemic and nonischemic heart failure patients. *PACE.* 2002;24:716.

282. St. John Sutton M, Plappert T, Young J, Hilpisch KE, Hill MRS. Cardiac resynchronization therapy results in improvement in echocardiographic parameters in heart failure patients with an indication for an ICD: evidence from the InSync trial. *PACE.* 2002;24:648. Abstract.

283. Strickberger SA for the AMIOVERT Trial Investigators. AMIOVERT is called a draw. www.theheart.org. November 15, 2000.

284. Swedberg K. Digoxin did not reduce mortality but reduced the rate of hospitalization due to worsening heart failure among patients with heart failure. *Evidence-based Cardiovasc Med.* 1997;1:44.

14

285. Swedberg K, Bergh CH, Dickstein K, McNay J, Steinberg M. The effects of moxonidine, a novel imidazoline, on plasma norepinephrine in patients with congestive heart failure. Moxonidine Investigators. *J Am Coll Cardiol.* 2000;35:398-404.

286. Swedberg K, Pfeffer M, Granger C, et al. Candesartan in heart failure—assessment of reduction in mortality and morbidity (CHARM): rationale and design. Charm-Programme Investigators. *J Card Fail* 1999;5:276-282.

287. Task Force of the Working Group on Heart Failure of the European Society of Cardiology. The treatment of heart failure. *Eur Heart J.* 1997;18:736-753.

288. Tierney WM, Overhage JM, Murray MD, et al. Effects of computerized guidelines for managing heart disease in primary care. *J Gen Intern Med.* 2003;18:967-976.

289. Torp-Pedersen C, Kober L. Effect of ACE inhibitor trandolapril on life expectancy of patients with reduced left-ventricular function after acute myocardial infarction. TRACE Study Group. Trandolapril Cardiac Evaluation. *Lancet.* 1999;354:9-12.

290. Torp-Pedersen C, Moller M, Bloch-Thomsen PE, et al. Dofetilide in patients with congestive heart failure and left ventricular dysfunction. Danish Investigations of Arrhythmia and Mortality on Dofetilide Study Group. *N Engl J Med.* 1999;341:857-865.

291. Torre-Amione G, Young JB, Colucci WS, Lewis BS, Kobrin I, Pratt CM, for the RITZ-II Trial Investigators. A prospective, randomized, double-blind, placebo-controlled, multicenter study of the safety and efficacy of tezosentan in patients with acute decompensated heart failure. Late-breaking clinical trials. Annual Scientific Sessions, American College of Cardiology, Orlando, Fla; March 2001.

292. Torree-Amione G, Young JB, Sastier F, et al. Immune modulation therapy reduces deaths and hospitalizations in class III/VI heart failure patients: results of a randomized clinical trial. *J Card Fail.* 2003;38:S10.

293. Tsuyuki RT, Ackman ML, Montague TJ. Effects of the 1994 Canadian Cardiovascular Society clinical practice guidelines for congestive heart failure. *Can J Cardiol.* 2002;18:147-152.

294. Tsuyuki RT, Yusuf S, Rouleau JL, et al. Combination neurohormonal blockade with ACE inhibitors, angiotensin II antagonists and beta-blockers in patients with congestive heart failure: design of the Randomized Evaluation of Strategies for Left Ventricular Dysfunction (RESOLVD) Pilot Study. *Can J Cardiol.* 1997;13:1166-1174.

295. Uretsky BF, Jessup M, Konstam MA, et al. Multicenter trial of oral enoximone in patients with moderate to moderately severe congestive heart failure. Lack of benefit compared with placebo. Enoximone Multicenter Trial Group. *Circulation*. 1990;82:774-780.

296. Uretsky BF, Thygesen K, Armstrong PW, et al. Acute coronary findings at autopsy in heart failure patients with sudden death: results from the assessment of treatment with lisinopril and survival (ATLAS) trial. *Circulation*. 2000;102:611-616.

297. Uretsky BF, Young JB, Shahidi FE, Yellen LG, Harrison MC, Jolly MK. Randomized study assessing the effect of digoxin withdrawal in patients with mild to moderate chronic congestive heart failure: results of the PROVED trial. PROVED Investigative Group. *J Am Coll Cardiol*. 1993;22:955-962.

298. VALIANT Investigators. Valsartan in acute myocardial infarction. International newsletter.

299. van Gilst WH, Kingma JH, Peels KH, Dambrink JH, St John Sutton M. Which patient benefits from early angiotensin-converting enzyme inhibition after myocardial infarction? Results of one-year serial echocardiographic follow-up from the Captopril and Thrombolysis Study (CATS). *J Am Coll Cardiol*. 1996;28:114-121.

300. van Veldhuisen DJ, Man in't Veld AJ, Dunselman PH, et al. Double-blind placebo-controlled study of ibopamine and digoxin in patients with mild to moderate heart failure: results of the Dutch Ibopamine Multicenter Trial (DIMT). *J Am Coll Cardiol*. 1993;22:1564-1573.

301. Waagstein F, Bristow MR, Swedberg K, et al. Beneficial effects of metoprolol in idiopathic dilated cardiomyopathy. Metoprolol in Dilated Cardiomyopathy (MDC) Trial Study Group. *Lancet*. 1993;342:1441-1446.

302. Waldo AL, Camm AJ, de Ruyter H, et al. Effect of d-sotalol on mortality in patients with left ventricular dysfunction after recent and remote myocardial infarction. The SWORD Investigators. Survival With Oral d-Sotalol. *Lancet*. 1996;348:7-12.

303. Wang TJ, Larson MG, Levy D, et al. Plasma natriuretic peptide levels and the risk of cardiovascular events and death. *N Engl J Med*. 2004;350:655-663.

304. Weber KT. Aldosterone and spironolactone in heart failure. *N Engl J Med*. 1999;341:753-755. Editorial.

305. Wever EF, Hauer RN, Van Capelle FJ, et al. Randomized study of implantable defibrillator as first-choice therapy versus conventional strategy in postinfarct sudden death survivors. *Circulation*. 1995;91:2195-2203.

14

306. Whellan DJ, Gaulden L, Gattis WA, et al. The benefit of implementing a heart failure disease management program. *Arch Intern Med.* 2001;161:2223-2228.

307. Wilkoff BL, Cook JR, Epstein AE, et al; Dual Chamber and VVI Implantable Defibrillator Trial Investigators. Dual-chamber pacing or ventricular backup pacing in patients with an implantable defibrillator: the Dual Chamber and VVI Implantable Defibrillator (DAVID) Trial. *JAMA.* 2002;288:3115-3123.

308. Wood MA, Brown-Mahoney C, Kay GN, et al. Clinical outcomes after ablation and pacing therapy for atrial fibrillation: a meta-analysis. *Circulation.* 2000;101:1138-1144.

309. The Xamoterol in Servere Heart Failure Study Group. Xamoterol in severe heart failure. *Lancet.* 1990;336:1-6.

310. Yancy CW, Chang SF. Clinical characteristics and outcomes in patients admitted with heart failure with preserved systolic function: a report from the ADHERE™ database. *J Card Fail.* 2003;9(suppl 5):S84. Abstract.

311. Yancy CW, Saltzberg M, Berkowitz RL, Horton DP, Silver MA; the FUSION Investigators. Management of patients with congestive heart failure after hospitalization: results from the follow up serial infusions of nesiritide (FUSION) trial. *J Card Fail.* 2003;9(suppl 1):S11.

312. Young JB. Assessment of heart failure. In: Colucci WS, Braunwald E, eds. *Atlas of Heart Diseases. Heart Failure: Cardiac Function and Dysfunction.* Vol. IV. Philadelphia, Pa: Current Medicine; 1995:7.1-7.19.

313. Young JB, Abraham WT. Effect of cardiac resynchronization on disease progression in patients with mild heart failure symptoms and an indication for an ICD—results of a randomized double blind study. *J Card Fail.* 2003;9(suppl 1):S11.

314. Young JB, Abraham WT, Liem L, Leon AR. Cardiac resynchronization therapy benefits patients with ICD indications—results of the InSync ICD trial. *PACE.* 2002;24:694. Abstract.

315. Young JB, Abraham WT, Smith AL, et al; Multicenter InSync ICD Randomized Clinical Evaluation (MIRACLE ICD) Trial Investigators. Combined cardiac resynchronization and implantable cardioversion defibrillation in advanced chronic heart failure: the MIRACLE ICD Trial. *JAMA.* 2003;289:2685-2694.

316. Young JB, Farmer JA. The diagnostic evaluation of patients with heart failure. In: Hosenpud JD, Greenberg BH, eds. *Congestive Heart Failure: Pathophysiology, Diagnosis, and Comprehensive Approach to Management.* New York, NY: Springer-Verlag; 1994:597-622.

317. Young JB, Gheorghiade M, Packer M, et al, on behalf of the PROVED and RADIANCE investigators. Are low serum levels of digoxin effective in chronic heart failure? Evidence challenging the accepted guidelines for a therapeutic serum level of the drug. *J Am Coll Cardiol.* 1993;21(suppl A):378A.

318. Young JB, Pratt CM. Hemodynamic and hormonal alterations in patients with heart failure: toward a contemporary definition of heart failure. *Semin Nephrol.* 1994;14:427-440.

319. Young JB, the VMAC Investigators. Vasodilator Management of Acute Congestive Heart Failure. *Late Breaking Clinical Trials.* American Heart Association; November 2000; New Orleans, La.

320. Young JB, Weiner DH, Yusuf S, et al. Patterns of medication use in patients with heart failure: a report from the registry of Studies of Left Ventricular Dysfunction (SOLVD). *South Med J.* 1994;88:514-523.

321. Yusuf S, Pfeffer MA, Swedberg K, et al; CHARM Investigators and Committees. Effects of candesartan in patients with chronic heart failure and preserved left-ventricular ejection fraction: the CHARM-Preserved Trial. *Lancet.* 2003;362:777-781.

322. Zannad F, Alla F, Dousset B, Perez A, Pitt B. Limitation of excessive extracellular matrix turnover may contribute to survival benefit of spironolactone therapy in patients with congestive heart failure: insights from the randomized aldactone evaluation study (RALES). Rales Investigators. *Circulation.* 2000;102:2700-2706.

323. Cleland JG, Daubert JC, Erdmann E, et al; CARE-HF study Steering Committee and Investigators. The CARE-HF study (CArdiac REsynchronisation in Heart Failure study): rationale, design and end-points. *Eur J Heart Fail.* 2001;3:481-489.

324. Sudden Cardiac Death in Heart Failure Trial (SCD-HeFT) Findings. Presented at American College of Cardiology Annual Scientific Session, New Orleans, La: 2004.

14

INDEX

15

356

15

15

15

364

15

15

15

370

15

373

15

375

15

15

15

15